FRCS Trauma and Orthopaedics Viva

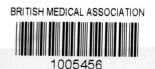

FRCS Trauma and Orthopaedics Viva

EDITED BY

Nev Davies FRCS (Tr&Orth)

Consultant in Trauma and Orthopaedics, The Royal Berkshire Hospital, Reading

Will Jackson FRCS (Tr&Orth)

Consultant, Nuffield Department of Orthopaedics, Rheumatology and Musculoskeletal Sciences, Oxford University, Oxford, UK

Andrew Price DPhil, FRCS (Tr&Orth)

Professor and Honorary Clincial Lecturer, Nuffield Department of Orthopaedics, Rheumatology and Musculoskeletal Sciences, Oxford University, Oxford, UK

Jonathan Rees MA, FRCS (Eng), MD, FRCS (Orth)

University Lecturer in Orthopaedic Surgery and Head of Education, Nuffield Department of Orthopaedics, Rheumatology and Musculoskeletal Sciences, Oxford University, Oxford, UK

Chris Lavy OBE, MD, MCh, FRCS

Professor and Honorary Clinical Lecturer, Nuffield Department of Orthopaedics, Rheumatology and Musculoskeletal Sciences, Oxford University, Oxford, UK

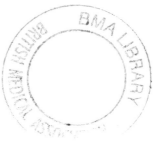

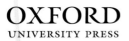

OXFORD
UNIVERSITY PRESS

OXFORD
UNIVERSITY PRESS

Great Clarendon Street, Oxford OX2 6DP
United Kingdom

Oxford University Press is a department of the University of Oxford.
It furthers the University's objective of excellence in research, scholarship,
and education by publishing worldwide. Oxford is a registered trade mark of
Oxford University Press in the UK and in certain other countries

© Oxford University Press 2012

The moral rights of the authors have been asserted

First Edition published in 2012
Impression: 3

British Library Cataloguing in Publication Data

Data available

Library of Congress Cataloging in Publication Data
Library of Congress Control Number: 2012934753

ISBN 978–0–19–964709–5

Printed and bound in Great Britain by Ashford Colour Press Ltd

Preface

In the surgical specialities we probably end up sitting more exams than any other profession. If you have purchased this book you are probably approaching the last serious exam that you will need to take. One of the problems is that it has now been several years since you sat a 'serious exam'. As such we are all at fault for building this next exam into something very big and very important, mainly because of the implications that failing has on both your professional and personal lives.

A number of your predecessors attended our clinical revision course in Oxford and one of the analogies we have always spoken about is being 'exam fit', the exam analogy to the sporting 'match fitness'. As it is several years since you have taken an exam it is important to practice in exam situations and also to practice structuring answers to exam questions. If you do this for the first time in the real exam you will struggle. If it had been several years since you stopped playing a sport you would want and need a few second-team games before making your return to the first team—the same is true for this exam. So having revised over the last year or so and having passed your written exam you should have a good amount of core knowledge, but your 'exam training' should now be about seeing lots of clinical cases, practising your short-case technique, and importantly not forgetting to practice your viva technique. A wise professor once told us to revise in the way one is going to be examined, and this revision book is designed to help you to do this.

There are times when you might find it useful to read this book alone, but it has really been designed to be used in small groups. The philosophy of our course has always been that in the lead up to this particular exam you learn as much from watching and listening to your colleagues answer viva questions (in fact probably more!) than when you are asked them directly yourself. This book is therefore set out in a simple format with a starting clinical photograph, radiograph, or diagram and a set of questions followed by some suggested answers on the next page. Just as in a normal exam, the questions get more detailed as you progress further into the viva. The book allows you to work alone, with a colleague, or even a team of colleagues who are taking the exam together.

During the viva exam it is quite easy to answer a seemingly difficult question (or even an easy question) in the wrong way and dig a very significant hole for yourself. It then becomes difficult to climb out of this hole; it affects your confidence and can have a detrimental effect on your performance. Remember, the examiners don't know you and you need to impress them with your safe, sensible, and knowledgeable approach to their questions. There are many different ways to start and respond to viva questions, and by watching and listening to a number of your colleagues answering these questions you will observe and learn that some methods are certainly safer than others. This book does not aim to tell you which methods to use, but working in groups allows further self-learning with regard to how you can plan to answer sensibly and safely, which is what your examiners are really looking for.

We hope you benefit from using this book; you are reminded that it is not a comprehensive knowledge text but an aid and approach to answering questions similar to the ones that you will encounter shortly in your exam. A final tip that we give to all candidates on our course is that when you are faced with that very very difficult clinical photograph or X-ray and you really have little idea of the very rare diagnosis before you, just 'say what you see'; this again reminds you that periods of silence in the exam do not score well but talking sensibly about what is in front of you will help you perform. We wish you the very best for your forthcoming exams and hard work now really does pay dividends for your future orthopaedic surgical career.

Nev Davies
Will Jackson
Andrew Price
Jonathan Rees
Chris Lavy

Acknowledgements

The editors and Oxford University Press would like to thank Paul Marks and FNS Publishing for the first publication of this book and their support. They would also like to thank Rachel Hubbard for her contribution to the first publication.

Contents

List of Contributors

Peter Burge FRCS
Consultant Hand Surgeon,
Nuffield Orthopaedic Centre, Oxford

Rachel Buckingham MB ChB, FRCS (Tr & Orth)
Orthopaedic Consultant,
Nuffield Orthopaedic Centre, Oxford

Jon Campion MBBS, BMedSci, FRCS
Consultant Orthopaedic Surgeon,
Northampton General Hospital, Northampton

Ramesh Chennagiri MS Orth, FRCS Orth, Dip Hand Surg (Br)
Consultant in Trauma & Orthopaedics,
Wycombe Hospital, High Wycombe

Paul Cooke MB ChM, FRCS
Consultant Orthopaedic Surgeon,
Nuffield Orthopaedic Centre, Oxford

Nev Davies BSc, FRCS (Tr & Orth)
Consultant Trauma & Orthopaedic Surgeon,
The Royal Berkshire Hospital, Reading

Mark Deakin MBBS, MSc, FRCS (Tr & Orth)
Consultant Trauma & Orthopaedic Surgeon,
The John Radcliffe Hospital, Oxford

Ad Gandhe BSc, MBBS, FRCS (Tr & Orth)
Consultant Trauma & Orthopaedic Surgeon,
Queen Alexandra Hospital, Portsmouth

Max Gibbons MA, FRCS
Consultant Orthopaedic Surgeon,
Nuffield Orthopaedic Centre, Oxford

Richie Gill BEng, DPhil
University Lecturer in Orthopaedic
Engineering & Group Head of the OOEC,
Botnar Research Centre, Nuffield Orthopaedic Centre, Oxford

Sion Glynn-Jones MA, DPhil, FRCS (Orth)
Senior Lecturer and Consultant Orthopaedic Surgeon,
Nuffield Orthopaedic Centre/ NDORMS, Oxford

Roger Gundle MA, DPhil, FRCS (Orth)
Consultant Orthopaedic Surgeon,
Nuffield Orthopaedic Centre, Oxford

Steve Gwilym DPhil, FRCS (Tr & Orth)
Clinical Lecturer in Orthopaedics,
Nuffield Orthopaedic Centre / NDORMS, Oxford

William Jackson FRCS (Tr & Orth)
Consultant Orthopaedic Surgeon,
Nuffield Orthopaedic Centre, Oxford

Chris Lavy OBE, MD MCh, FRCS
Hon Consultant Orthopaedic Surgeon,
Nuffield Orthopaedic Centre / NDORMS, Oxford

Paul Marks BA, LLM, MD, FRCS
Consultant Spine/Neurosurgeon,
Leeds General Infirmary, Leeds

Rebecca Mills BA, BMBCh
Senior House Officer,
Royal Berkshire Hospital, Reading

David Noyes FRCS (Tr & Orth)
Consultant Trauma Surgeon,
The John Radcliffe Hospital, Oxford

Andrew Price MA, DPhil, FRCS (Orth)
Professor of Orthopaedic Surgery and Consultant Orthopaedic Surgeon,
Nuffield Orthopaedic Centre/NDORMS, Oxford

Jonathan Rees MA, MBBS, FRCS (Eng), MD, FRCS (Orth)
University Lecturer in Orthopaedics and Consultant Shoulder & Elbow Surgeon,
Head of Education, Director Oxford Orthopaedic & Simulatoin Centre,
Nuffield Orthopaedic Centre / NDORMS, Oxford

Jeremy Reynolds FRCS (Tr & Orth), MB ChB, BSc (Hons)
Consultant Orthopaedic Surgeon,
Nuffield Orthopaedic Centre, Oxford

Bob Sharp BMBCh, MA, FRCS (Tr & Orth)
Consultant Orthopaedic Surgeon,
Nuffield Orthopaedic Centre, Oxford

Aman Sharma MBBS, MRCSEd, MPhil (Cantab), MRCS
Spinal Research Fellow,
Nuffield Orthopaedic Centre, Oxford

Tim Theologis MSc, PhD, FRCS
Consultant Orthopaedic Surgeon,
Nuffield Orthopaedic Centre, Oxford

Dionysios Trigkilidas BSc (Hons), MBBS, MRCS
Registrar in Trauma & Orthopaedics,
Watford General Hospital, Watford

Andrew Wainwright FRCS (Tr & Orth)
Consultant Orthopaedic Surgeon,
Nuffield Orthopaedic Centre, Oxford

Nick Ward MbChB, FRCS (Tr & Orth)
Consultant Trauma & Orthopaedic Surgeon,
Frimley Park Hospital, Frimley

Viva Table 1

Hands and Paediatric Orthopaedics

Section 1 Hands

Viva 1

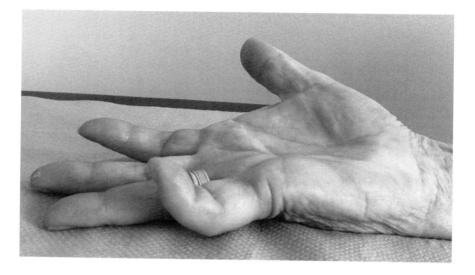

What is the likely diagnosis?

What are the risk factors for this condition?

What are the two main components seen in the histology of mature tissue from this condition?

What are the management options?

What are the risks of surgical treatment?

What is the likely diagnosis?

The clinical photograph shows flexion of the right little finger metacarpophalangeal (MCP) joint, suggestive of Dupuytren's contracture.

What are the risk factors for this condition?

The risk factors associated with Dupuytren's disease include: positive family history; liver disease; high alcohol intake; diabetes mellitus, and epilepsy.

What are the two main components seen in the histology of mature tissue from this condition?

Classic histological appearance is the presence of myofibroblast cells (probably derived from fibroblasts) and thick collagen fibres.

What are the management options?

The management options are non-operative measures and operative procedures.

Non-operative options include observation (and possibly splintage, especially at night).

Some authors have reported that steroid injections to early palmar nodules may reduce local tenderness. Although promising short-term results have been reported with collagenase injection, no long-term results are available.

Surgical options include:

- Percutaneous fasciotomy, especially for mild contractures affecting MCP joint contractures
- Segmental/palmar fasciectomy
- Regional fasciectomy (and Z-plasty closure or skin grafting)
- Dermo-fasciectomy and skin grafting
- Proximal interphalangeal (PIP) joint arthrodesis (for severe or recurrent disease)
- Occasionally, amputation of the digit (for severe or recurrent disease)

What are the risks of surgical treatment?

Specific surgical risks include:

- Delayed wound healing, infection
- Tendon, nerve, and vessel injury
- Temporary or permanent numbness
- Necrosis of the digit and amputation
- Incomplete correction
- Recurrence and re-operation
- Joint stiffness
- Reduced flexion/extension especially at the PIP joint
- Pain, swelling, and tenderness; occasionally chronic regional pain syndrome

Viva 2

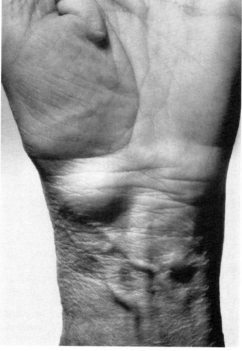

Reproduced from C. Bulstrode et al., Oxford Textbook of Trauma and Orthopaedics second edition, 2011, figure 6.13.2, page 512, with permission from Oxford University Press.

What is the likely diagnosis of the cystic, soft-tissue lump shown in the photograph? From what structure does it commonly arise?

What clinical test, outpatient procedure, and simple imaging investigation can be performed to confirm the diagnosis?

Give a histological definition of this condition.

What are the other sites for these cystic swellings in the wrist and hand?

How would you manage this condition in a 26-year-old woman who works as a secretary and presents to you for the first time?

What is the risk of recurrence post-excision?

What is the likely diagnosis of the cystic, soft-tissue lump shown in the photograph? From what structure does it commonly arise?

The appearance of the lump at the wrist is suggestive of a ganglion cyst. Approximately two-thirds of such cysts originate in the radiocarpal joint. The remaining third arise from the scapho-trapezoid joint.

What clinical test, outpatient procedure, and simple imaging investigation can be performed to confirm the diagnosis?

Clinical test = compressible lump which trans-illuminates

Outpatient procedure = aspiration of the ganglion under local anaesthetic

Simple imaging investigation = ultrasound scan

Give a histological definition of this condition.

A ganglion cyst is a fluid-filled cavity lined by compressed collagen and a few cells.

What are the other sites for these cystic swellings in the wrist and hand?

1. Ganglia in the hand are commonly seen over the dorsum of the wrist where they commonly arise from scapholunate ligament
2. Cysts arising from the distal interphalangeal (DIP) joint present as dorsal cysts and are called dorsal distal ganglia, mucoid, or mucous cysts
3. Smaller, firmer cysts may be found in relation to the flexor tendon sheath in the region of the A2 pulley. These are called palmar digital ganglia, flexor sheath ganglia, or pearl ganglia

Interosseous ganglia are uncommon, but when present are often in the lunate bone.

How would you manage this condition in a 26-year-old woman who works as a secretary and presents to you for the first time?

I would explain:

1. That a ganglion is a common benign cyst
2. That during the natural history of a ganglion it can often fluctuate in size periodically and may resolve spontaneously if simply observed
3. Treatment options and their potential risks include:
   - Simple observation (few if any risks)
   - Aspiration of the cyst (small risks of haematoma or infection, radial artery damage, and recurrence)
   - Surgical excision of the ganglion, open or arthroscopic (risks of anaesthesia and surgery including nerve, vessel, and tendon injury, haematoma and infection, pain, swelling, tenderness, stiffness, and recurrence)

What is the risk of recurrence post-excision?

The risk of recurrence in some published series is similar for all three treatment options above, so observation is the safe course of action.

Viva 3

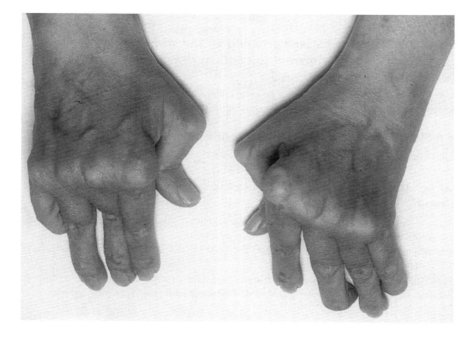

Describe the picture.

How would you grade the thumb condition radiologically?

Why does subluxation occur in this condition?

How could you explain the hyperextension deformity of the MCP joint?

What are the management options?

How would you treat this patient who has unremitting carpo-metacarpal (CMC) joint pain despite full non-operative treatment and who is fit for surgery?

What are the advantages and disadvantages and surgical risks with simple excision arthroplasty?

Describe the picture

This is a clinical photo of the dorsal aspect of the hands showing a symmetrical, deforming, polyarthropathy consistent with rheumatoid arthritis. There are bilateral Z-shaped thumbs, swan-necking of the right middle finger, and marked ulnar deviation of all fingers at the MCP joints.

How would you grade the thumb condition radiologically?

I would use the Eaton and Littler system to stage this condition.

- Stage I—joint space widening, normal articular contours
- Stage II—up to one-third subluxation (on stress radiographs, thumbs resting on plate and pushing against each other): osteophytes < 2 mm, scapho-trapezio-trapezoidal (STT) joint is normal
- Stage III—marked narrowing of joint space, more than one-third subluxation: osteophytes > 2 mm
- Stage IV—pan-trapezial arthritis

Why does subluxation occur in this condition?

The palmar oblique ligament (also known as the 'beak' ligament) is a very strong ligament extending from the trapezium to the base of the first metacarpal. Degenerative attenuation and rupture of this ligament results in dorsal subluxation of the first metacarpal.

How could you explain the hyperextension deformity of the MCP joint?

Dorsal subluxation of the CMC joint causes metacarpal adduction, a thumb in the palm deformity, and reduction in thumb span. This leads to a secondary compensatory hyperextension at the MCP joint in an effort to increase the thumb span.

What are the management options?

Non-operative options include: oral analgesia; activity modification; use of splints; physiotherapy; and intra-articular steroid injection which could be performed in the outpatient clinic or under fluoroscopic guidance.

Operative options include:

1. Excision of the trapezium offers satisfactory pain relief in most cases and preserves movement. Results are reliable. However, pinch grip may be weakened
2. The addition of a suspension procedure and tendon interposition has been shown to offer no extra benefit
3. Implant arthroplasty has failed to offer good long-term results and early implant failure has made this procedure less popular
4. Rarely, CMC arthrodesis is performed in young adult manual workers as this procedure offers a stable thumb with good pinch grip. However, the manoeuvrability of the thumb is affected
5. First metacarpal-basal osteotomy may be considered, especially in earlier stages of the disease

How would you treat this patient who has unremitting CMC joint pain despite full non-operative treatment and who is fit for surgery?

I would offer this patient excision of the trapezium and fusion of the MCP joint under general anaesthetic (GA)/regional block. I would perform the procedure as a day-case.

What are the advantages and disadvantages and surgical risks with simple excision arthroplasty?

Trapezium excision results in good pain relief and consequently improved function, but slight shortening of the thumb can cause reduced power of pinch. Risks specific to the procedure include painful scar, infection, nerve damage (superficial branch of the radial nerve), blood vessel damage (radial artery), incomplete relief of symptoms (especially if adjacent joints are affected by osteoarthritis), a relatively slow recovery of function and attainment of maximal pain relief, and instability of the carpus.

Viva 4

A 20-year-old man presents 48 h after he was involved in a fight with another person, when he sustained a punching injury shown in the photograph below.

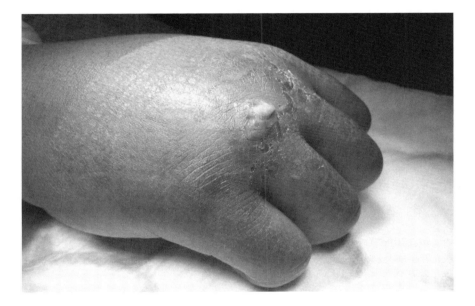

What is the likely nature of this injury?

How would you assess this patient?

How would you treat this injury?

Which organisms commonly cause infection with this type of injury?

Which antibiotics would you use to cover these organisms?

What is the likely nature of this injury?

There is a 'fight-bite' puncture wound over the right ring finger MCP joint that may have been caused by a penetrating human tooth and may extend into the joint causing cartilage injury, bony fracture, and associated joint infection ± osteomyelitis.

How would you assess this patient?

I would take a full history including the circumstances of the injury, past medical history, and tetanus immunization status. I would look for systemic signs such as fever and tachycardia. On local examination, I would look for signs of cellulitis, tendon sheath infection, tendon rupture, and septic arthritis. I would request plain radiographs to exclude the presence of a foreign body and a fracture. I would also request baseline blood tests [full blood count (FBC), erythrocyte sedimentation rate (ESR) and C-reactive protein (CRP)].

How would you treat this injury?

My initial treatment would be to provide tetanus prophylaxis if indicated and apply sterile dressing to cover the wound. I would withhold antibiotics, if systemically well, until tissue samples are obtained.

I would take the patient to theatre for urgent debridement under GA with a tourniquet around the arm. During surgery, I would obtain pus swab and tissue samples for histology and microbiological examination. I would extend the wound and look for tendon damage (re-create fist by flexing the MCP joint). If the tendon is ruptured, I would tag the tendon ends and not attempt primary repair. I would inspect the joint. I would then wash the wound with copious amounts of fluid. I would leave the wound open and apply a splint over non-adhesive dressing. I would commence broad-spectrum antibiotics, pending culture results and arrange for a further look after 48 h.

Which organism commonly causes infection with this type of injury?

Although *Eikenella corrodens* is peculiar to this injury, *Staphylococcus aureus* is the commonest organism; anaerobic bacteria may also be implicated.

Which antibiotics would you use to cover these organisms?

I would prescribe broad-spectrum antibiotics according to local microbiological protocols such as co-amoxiclav, cephalosporin, and metronidazole.

Viva 5

A 24-year-old male cyclist has been knocked off his bicycle sustaining an isolated injury to his left wrist.

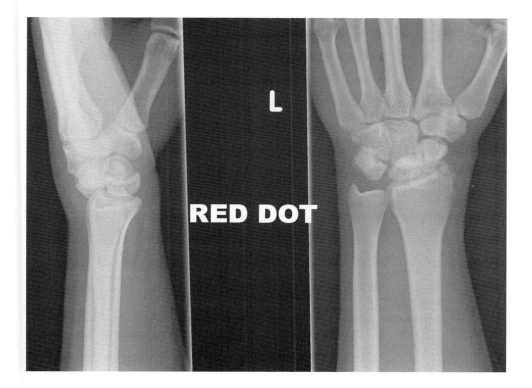

Describe the appearances of these radiographs.

How would you classify this injury?

How would you assess this patient's isolated injury?

How would you manage this injury initially and definitively?

Describe the appearances of these radiographs

Postero-anterior (PA) and lateral radiographs of the left wrist showing a perilunate dislocation.

PA view shows:

1. Disruption of the 'Gilula's' smooth carpal lines that join the proximal joint surfaces of the proximal row of carpal bones at the radiocarpal joint and the distal joint surfaces of the proximal row of carpal bones and the proximal joint surfaces of the distal row of carpal bones (at the mid-carpal joint). The Capitate appears to overlap the lunate
2. Hyperflexion of the scaphoid (scaphoid signet ring sign)
3. Abnormal triangular appearance of the lunate, but lunate located in the lunate fossa of the radius
4. Overlapping of the lunate and triquetrum [unable to visualize lunotriquetral (LT) joint]
5. No obvious fractures of radial styloid, scaphiod, capitate, triquetrum, hamate, or ulnar styloid.

Lateral view shows:

1. Dorsal dislocation of the capitate head from its articulation with the lunate at the mid carpal joint and dorsal translation of distal carpal row and metacarpals relative to the long axis of the radius.

How would you classify this injury?

Perilunate injuries often follow a typical pattern as described by Mayfield. Assuming there are indeed no fractures, this is a 'lesser arc' ligament-rupturing perilunate dislocation. 'Greater arc' injuries also include one or more fractures, typically of the radial styloid, scaphoid, capitate, hamate, triquetrum (± ulnar styloid). A typical lesser arc perilunate injury follows the 'Mayfield sequence' of ligament failures in sequential defined stages:

Check:

Stage I: failure of the radiocarpal ligament
Stage II: failure of the scapholunate ligament
Stage III: failure of the LT ligament and dorsal mid-carpal dislocation
Stage IV: palmar dislocation of lunate at the radiocarpal joint

Therefore this patient's injury is a Mayfield stage III lesser arc perilunate dislocation.

How would you assess this patient's isolated injury?

I would take a detailed history including handedness, occupation, mechanism of injury, co-morbidities, and time since last meal. I would examine carefully for abnormal wrist contour, pain and swelling, and signs of median nerve compression, and document median nerve function, sensory, and motor function.

How would you manage this injury initially and definitively?

Initial management

- Exclude another injury. Provide analgesia. Regular neurovascular observations
- Keep nil-by-mouth [± intravenous (IV) hydration if necessary]
- Splintage [e.g. padded plaster of Paris (POP) slap + loose bandage]
- High elevation (Bradford sling or Chinese finger traps)
- Explain severity of injury to patient
- Prepare and consent patient for urgent theatre
- Minimum initial intervention requires closed (± open) reduction of the dislocation using image intensifier control (± carpal tunnel decompression) + POP slab stabilization

Definitive intervention (± specialist hand surgery advice)

- Would include closed but anatomical restoration of carpal alignment using joystick k-wires (arthroscopically and image intensifier controlled) + buried k-wire stabilization of scapholunate, LT, and mid-carpal joints
- OR open dorsal anatomical carpal reduction, buried k-wire stabilization, and repair of scapholunate, LT, dorsal and palmar radiocarpal, ligaments
- Post-operatively: high elevation and careful neurovascular observation. Full POP for 2 weeks. Removal of wires at 8 weeks and mobilization
- Risks of post-traumatic carpal instability or stiffness ± osteoarthritis

Viva 6

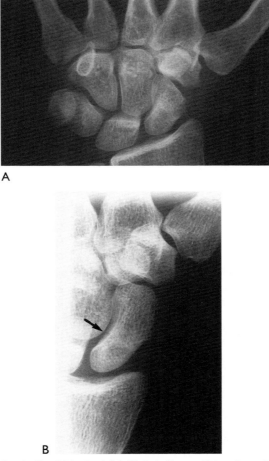

A

B

Describe these radiographs and explain the diagnosis.

What are the indications for internal fixation of scaphoid fractures?

Should acute non-displaced fractures be fixed?

What are the complications of this injury?

How would you plan the management of an established non-union of a scaphoid fracture?

Describe these radiographs and explain the diagnosis

The standard PA radiograph of the wrist does not show any obvious fractures; however, there is a subtle, non-displaced fracture of the scaphoid visible on the scaphoid view. This view is obtained by putting the hand and wrist in ulnar deviation, along with 15° of cephalad angulation of the X-ray tube.

What are the indications for internal fixation of scaphoid fractures?

Indications for internal fixation of a scaphoid fracture are:

1. If the displacement is more than 1 mm
2. Or the scapholunate angle > 60°
3. Lunocapitate angle >15°
4. Intrascaphoid angle > 20° (dorsal humpback)
5. Proximal pole fractures, fractures associated with a peri-lunate dislocation
6. Delayed union

Should acute non-displaced fractures be fixed?

The overall rate of non-union scaphoid fractures treated in POP is 10%.

Not all acute non-displaced fractures need fixation, although there are some advantages. Studies have shown better early outcome scores, grip strength, and range of motion (ROM) with fixation but no difference after 12–16 weeks. The rate of delayed union has been shown to be less with early fixation. Patients should be advised to avoid cigarette smoking to optimize their potential for bone healing.

What are the complications of this injury?

The two major complications related to this injury are avascular necrosis (AVN)of the proximal pole and non-union.

How would you plan the management of an established non union of a scaphoid fracture?

If arthritic changes are not present on the radiographs, fixation with bone graft should be attempted in an effort to get the fracture to unite. Zaidemberg and colleagues have reported excellent (100% union in 11 patients) results with a vascularized distal radial bone graft based on the 1,2 intermeta-carpal branch of the radial artery. More recent studies have reported a success rate of around 70%. If arthritic changes are present and patient is symptomatic, salvage procedures such as radial styloid-ectomy, proximal row carpectomy, scaphoid excision, and four-corner fusion and arthrodesis of the wrist should be considered.

Viva 7

This adolescent man comes to your clinic complaining of non-specific wrist pain and a magnetic resonance imaging (MRI) scan he has obtained privately.

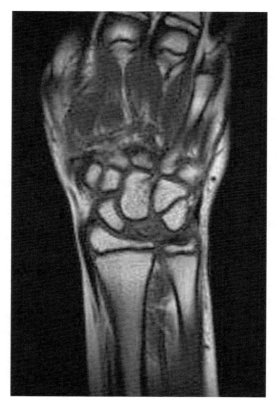

Reproduced from C. Bulstrode et al., Oxford Textbook of Trauma and Orthopaedics second edition, 2011, figure 13.23.7, p. 1617, with permission from Oxford University Press.

Describe what you see in the image.

What is the cause of this condition?

What is the staging system for this condition?

What else should you look for on the radiographs?

What are the management options?

Describe what you see in the image

This T1 magnetic resonance image shows low signal density in the lunate, suggestive of Keinbock's disease.

What is the cause of this condition?

Kienbock's disease is AVN of the lunate bone in the wrist.

What is the staging system for this condition?

The Lichtmann classification, which recognizes four stages:

Stage I: normal radiographs, possible stress fractures

Stage II: sclerosis of the lunate, no collapse

Stage IIIA: fragmentation and early collapse

Stage IIIB: IIIA + scapholanate dissociation and fixed rotation of the scaphoid

Stage IV: IIIB + degenerative changes in the wrist joint

What else should you look for on the radiographs?

I would look for negative ulnar variance on antero-posterior (AP) radiographs taken with the forearm in mid-prone position.

What are the management options?

The condition can be managed non-operatively with analgesia and splintage. Operative options include joint levelling procedures (radius shortening), wrist denervation, partial or total wrist fusion, and proximal row carpectomy. Choice of treatment depends on the stage of the disease, degree of symptoms, and patient factors.

Viva 8

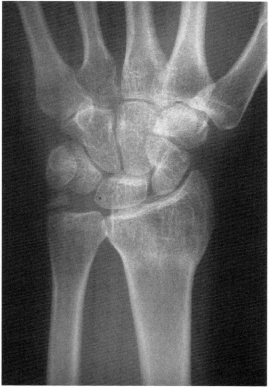

Reproduced from C. Bulstrode et al., Oxford Textbook of Trauma and Orthopaedics second edition, 2011, figure 6.4.9, p. 440, with permission from Oxford University Press.

Describe what you see on this radiograph of a 22-year-old with ulnar-sided wrist pain.

Which soft tissue structure would you expect to be involved?

Can you simplify the anatomy of this complex structure?

What are the management options for this condition?

Describe what you see on this radiograph of a 22-year-old with ulnar-sided wrist pain

This AP radiograph of the wrist shows ulnar positive variance. This appearance is typical of ulnar abutment syndrome.

Which soft tissue structure would you expect to be involved?

Triangular fibrocartilage complex (TFCC) tears are frequently associated with this condition (Class 2 lesion).

Can you simplify the anatomy of this complex structure?

The TFCC is a pyramid-shaped fibrocartilagenous ligamentous structure found at the distal aspect of the ulna.

It comprises a fibrocartilagenous disc (a meniscus-like structure) and a sling of ligaments and acts as a key stabilizer of the distal radioulnar (DRU) joint and the ulnocarpal joint.

What are the management options for this condition?

Non-operative measures are splint, analgesia, and avoidance of aggravating activities. Operative options include arthroscopic wafer resection of ulna, or open ulnar shortening osteotomy.

Viva 9

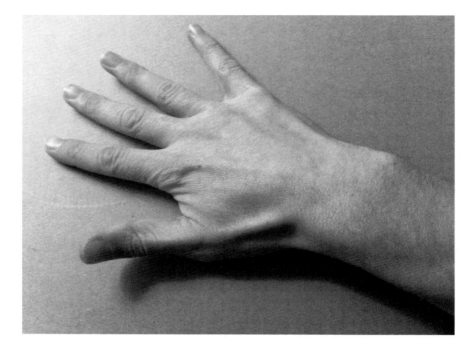

Tell me about the dorsal compartments at the wrist joint.

What is de Quervain's syndrome?

What are the clinical signs of de Quervain's syndrome?

What are the management options for de Quervain's syndrome?

What are the adverse effects of local steroid injection?

What are the pitfalls of surgery?

Tell me about the dorsal compartments at the wrist joint

There are six compartments in which the extensor tendons traverse the dorsum of the wrist

1. APL, EPB (abductor pollicis longus, extensor pollicis brevis)
2. ECRL, ECRB (extensor carpi radialis longus, extensor carpi radialis brevis)
3. EPL (extensor pollicis longus)
4. EI, EDC (extensor indicis, extensor digitorum communis)
5. EDM (extensor digiti minimi)
6. ECU (extensor carpi ulnaris)

What is de Quervain's syndrome?

It is a painful condition affecting the first compartment tendons of the wrist joint. It is commoner in females, especially post-partum.

What are the clinical signs of de Quervain's syndrome?

There is localized tenderness and/or swelling along the radial aspect of the wrist over APL/EPB. The Finkelstein test is considered positive if pain is elicited on holding the thumb and quickly ulnar-deviating the wrist. Pain may also be elicited on ulnar-deviating the wrist with fingers flexed over the thumb held in the palm.

What are the management options for de Quervain's syndrome?

Non-operative options are splintage, analgesia, and local steroid injection. If non-operative measures fail, surgical release could be considered. The procedure is done under GA or regional anaesthetic and with a upper arm tourniquet. Release may be achieved thorough a longitudinal or transverse skin incision.

What are the adverse effects of local steroid injection?

Adverse effects of local steroid injection are infection, skin atrophy and depigmentation, subcutaneous fat atrophy at the site of injection, injury to the superficial branch of radial nerve (painful neuroma), and tendon rupture.

What are the pitfalls of surgery?

Failure to recognize anatomical variation (EPB may lie in a separate compartment) may lead to incomplete relief of symptoms. Injury to the sensory branch of the radial nerve could result in a painful neuroma.

Viva 10

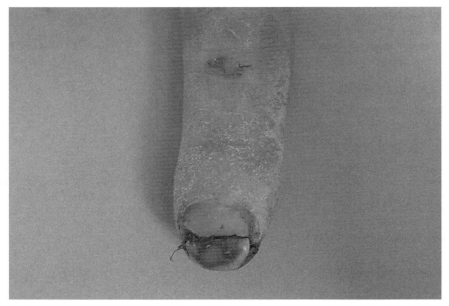

How would you manage this crush injury?

What would you explain to the patient?

How would you manage this crush injury?

I would take a relevant history, including: handedness; occupation; mechanism of injury; and co-morbidities. I will provide tetanus prophylaxis (if indicated) and antiseptic (betadine) dressing.

I would obtain radiographs to exclude an underlying fracture.

As definitive management, I would explore and repair the nail bed under local anaesthesia (digital block) and digital tourniquet.

The salient steps of the procedure are:

1. Remove the nail plate carefully
2. Inspect the nail bed and wash thoroughly
3. Copious lavage of any underlying fracture
4. Reduce fracture if present and stabilize (axial k-wire; remove after 3–4 weeks) if necessary
5. Repair nail bed with a 6-0 absorbable suture (VICRYL Rapide)
6. Wash and replace nail plate. Figure-of-eight stitch (or equivalent) to hold the nail plate in place

What would you explain to the patient?

I would explain that the nail plate will fall off and be gradually replaced by a new one, which may initially appear disfigured. There is a risk of some long-term nail deformity and discomfort in the region of the nail bed and some distal interphalangeal joint stiffness.

Viva Table 1

Hands and Paediatric Orthopaedics

Section 2 Paediatric Orthopaedics

Viva 11

This 2½-year-old girl is referred to your clinic with a limp.

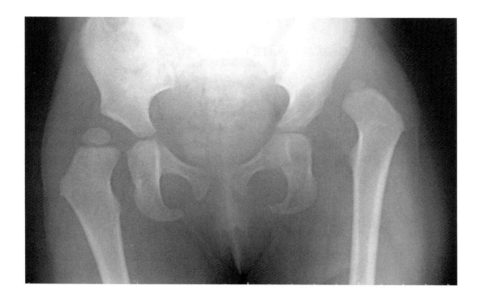

Describe the radiographic findings.

How would you proceed in your management from here?

What open operative approaches would you use to reduce this hip?

Describe the radiographic findings.

This is an AP pelvic radiograph showing a dislocated left hip and dysplastic acetabulum. Shenton's line is broken and the femoral head lies lateral and superior to the inferiomedial quadrant (made by the intersection of Perkin's and Hilgenreiner's lines).

How would you proceed in you management from here?

I would take a full history and examine the child. There may be risk factors for developmental dysplasia of the hip (DDH) including positive family history and/or decreased intrauterine space [first born, breech, oligohydramnios (associated packaging problems)].

More importantly I would be looking to see if there were any underlying neuromuscular conditions such as spina bifida, arthrogryphosis, or cerebral palsy. Examination may reveal a Trendelenberg gait, leg length discrepancy, fixed flexion deformity as well as reduced abduction of the left hip, which is the most consistent and reliable clinical sign of this condition.

I would organize an examination under anaesthesia (EUA) and arthrogram to delineate the anatomy of the acetabulum, soft tissues, and proximal femur. It would be unlikely that this hip would reduce closed. Blocks to reduction would include: an inverted limbus; elongated ligamentum teres; hour-glass constriction of the capsule; psoas tendon and pulvinar. Indications for open reduction include: failure of closed reduction; an unstable reducible hip, or soft tissue interposition preventing a congruent reduction.

What open operative approaches would you use to reduce this hip?

I would use a modified anterior (ilio-femoral) approach to the hip. I would place my skin incision parallel and distal to the iliac crest, passing 2 cm distal to the anterior superior iliac spine (ASIS) and extending medially within the groin skin crease.

I would identify and protect the lateral cutaneous nerve of the thigh and then distally I would develop the internervous plane between tensor fascia lata (superior gluteal nerve) and sartorius (femoral nerve). Splitting the iliac crest apophysis I would elevate the muscles en masse on both sides of the pelvis down to the sciatic notch and the superior border of the acetabulum. I would divide the straight head of rectus femoris and then make a T-shaped capsular incision to enter the hip joint and clear the acetabulum of pulvinar and redundant ligamentum teres (not the labrum). Any inverted labrum will require to be everted and one or more radial cuts may be necessary to allow this. The inferior capsule may also require release, with care not to damage the blood supply to the femoral head. It is likely there would be tightness in the iliopsoas and its tendon will need releasing to be able to reduce the hip.

I would then assess the need for: (1) a shortening femoral osteotomy and/or (2) pelvic osteotomy (e.g. Salter) to give more cover.

I would then perform a double-breasted capsular repair, close in layers and apply a hip spica cast with the hip in approximately 30° of abduction and internal rotation. The spica would need changing at 6 weeks for a total of 3 months. Post-operatively I would watch carefully for spica syndrome and organize an MRI scan to check that the hip remains enlocated.

The patient would require long-term follow-up to check that the hip develops normally.

Viva 12

This is a photograph of a 7-year-old girl sitting in a comfortable position. Her mother is concerned because she walks with her feet turned in.

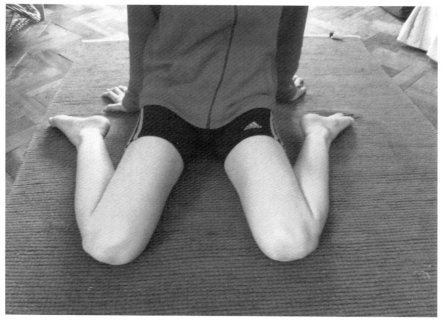

Photograph courtesy of Paul Thornton-Bott FRCS (Tr&Orth).

How would you proceed with your assessment?

You find on your examination that the child has extremely lax ligaments and increased internal rotation of both hips.

How do you grade ligamentous laxity in children?

The mother has asked about surgical treatment for this condition. What would you offer her?

How would you proceed with your assessment?

This clinical photograph shows a child sitting in the 'W' position.

Important questions in the history would include enquiry about the pregnancy and birth, developmental milestones, family history, and any significant past medical history. I would ask the child and the parents about current symptoms and concerns. The common causes of an in-toeing gait include metatarsus adductus, internal tibial torsion, and persistent femoral anteversion.

In the examination it is important to rule out asymmetry in the lower legs or any neurological signs, which could indicate an underlying spinal abnormality or neurological problem.

I would examine the gait (with shoes on and barefoot), looking specifically at the foot progression angle (negative in this case: normal is −5° to +20°)

With the child lying prone I would assess the torsional profile, looking for:

- Metatarsus adductus: foot shape in relation to heel bisector line
- Tibial torsion: thigh–foot angle (normal range 0–20°) if foot shape is normal or transmalleolar axis (normal range 0–45°) if foot is abnormal. Tibial torsion is defined as the angle between the transcondylar axis of the proximal tibia and the bi-malleolar axis (normal range 10–25° external)
- Femoral anteversion: range of motion, internal rotation (IR) > 60° (normal range 20–60°) > external rotation (ER) < 20° (normal range 30–60°); Ruwe's method, measure angle from vertical [finger on greater trochanter (GT), most lateral point; normal is about 8–14°]

I would also examine the spine and lower limb neurology as well as assess the degree of ligamentous laxity.

How do you grade ligamentous laxity in children?

I would use the Beighton score (out of 9):

Increased finger hyperextension—2 points
Increased thumb hyperextension—2 points
Increased elbow hyperextension—2 points (1 point for each side)
Increased knee hyperextension—2 points
Ability to place palms on floor with legs straight—1 point

The mother has asked about surgical treatment for this condition. What would you offer her?

This child's in-toeing gait is most likely due to persistent femoral anteversion which is a common cause in children older than 3 years.

I would reassure the mother that her daughter is physiologically normal but just at one end of the normal spectrum for children of her age. She may be interested to learn that the only effective treatment is to cut the femora, rotate them, and then fix them, which is a major surgical procedure, with risks, for essentially a cosmetic problem.

I would also explain the natural history of the condition that it tends to improve over the first decade but she may well be left in-toeing as an adult. As muscle balance improves into adulthood it rarely presents a functional problem.

Viva 13

This 13-year-old boy presented with pain in his right knee.

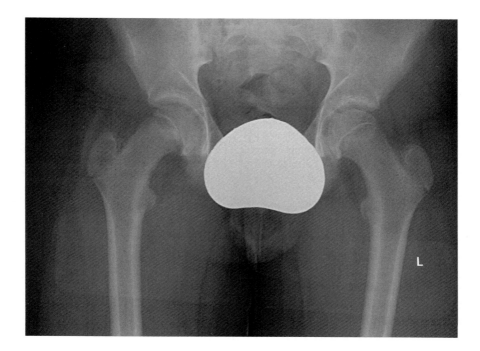

Describe the radiograph.

How do you classify this condition?

What is your management plan now with the right hip?

What is your management plan now with the left hip?

Describe the radiograph.

This is an AP radiograph of the pelvis in a skeletally immature child. There is a mild slip of the right upper femoral epiphysis (SUFE) with a positive Trethowan's sign. This is shown by drawing Klein's line up the lateral border of the femoral neck and noting it does not intersect the epiphysis.

How do you classify this condition?

I would use Loder's classification which divides SUFEs into stable and unstable based on the patient's ability to bear weight secondary to pain, and is important for predicting the risk of AVN. Other classifications grade the slip into mild (<33%), moderate (33–50%), or severe (>50%) the degree of which corresponds to the slip angle; this is useful when working out which are pinnable or not *in situ*.

What is your management plan now with the right hip?

I would take a full history for the patient and parents and examine the child. I am looking for any underlying cause for this SUFE such as endocrinopathy.

Examination findings would reveal classically a hip that externally rotates and abducts with flexion.

My management plan would consist of pinning this slip *in situ* with a single cannulated screw—use of more than one screw increases complications including AVN and chondrolysis.

I would perform this under GA on a fracture table, but would not use a forced reduction manoeuvre or traction which could increase the risk of AVN. I would use a triangulation technique to define the appropriate location for the skin incision. The thread of the screw should be in the centre of the epiphysis passing through perpendicular to the physis (this avoids perforating the femoral head). As the slip is usually postero-medial this technique usually requires an anterior femoral neck entry point. A minimum of two to three screw threads should pass into the epiphysis, depending on the size of the child and the instrumentation used.

What is your management plan now with the left hip?

Contralateral prophylactic screw fixation to prevent slip in the future remains a controversial topic. Options are to treat every case with contralateral fixation, versus pinning only those children thought to be at higher risk of contralateral slip or significant leg length discrepancy (less than 10 years old, underlying endocrinopathy).

Viva 14

This 8-month-old baby was brought to casualty with the above injury.

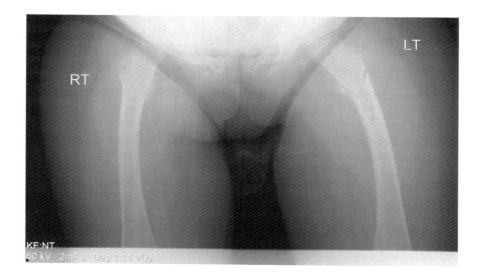

What are your thoughts?

Tell me about non-accidental injury and what you would do if you suspected it?

How would you treat this fracture?

What are your thoughts?

This is a AP view radiograph of a child's lower pelvis and femurs showing an oblique fracture at the left subtrochanteric level. I would like to take a detailed history from the parents or carer, as a fracture of the femur in a non-ambulant child could be a non-accidental injury (NAI). **You must pick this possibility up—it is reasonable for this to be a pass/fail type question.**

Tell me about non-accidental injury and what you would do if you suspected it.

Non-accidental injury is an injury deliberately inflicted by a parent or a caregiver. It may be difficult to suspect a parent or carer of abuse but we have a duty of care as professionals to ensure care and protection of children.

Child abuse itself can take different forms (physical, neglect, sexual, emotional, Munchausen's by proxy—rare): most are in combination. It is the second most common cause of death in young children (after trauma). Risk factors include first born, premature babies, stepchildren, family history of abuse, and parental IV drug abuse.

Firstly it is important to get the child into a safe environment and treat the traumatic injuries appropriately in the same way as for an accidental injury, according to Advanced Trauma Life Support (ATLS) guidelines and being mindful that there may be other more life-threatening injuries (subdural haematoma and 'shaken baby' syndrome). Having taken a detailed history from the parents and examined the child fully (with a chaperone), I would document my findings carefully in the notes. Clues suggesting NAI in the clinical assessment include a history that doesn't fit the injury, inconsistent explanations and delayed presentation, bruising patterns on the child, and retinal haemorrhages. I would inform the paediatricians of my concern about a possible NAI and make arrangements for the child to be admitted.

Radiographic clues for NAI include metaphyseal bucket handle corner fractures (virtually pathognomonic), rib fractures, and fractures of varying ages evidenced by different stages of healing.

How would you treat this fracture?

I would treat this fracture in gallows traction with a radiograph at 2–3 weeks, to show callus formation, and then gentle mobilization as comfort allows. A hip spica is sometimes used.

Viva 15

A 3-year-old child is referred from casualty with a 24-h history of fever, malaise, and reluctance to bear weight on his right leg.

What is your approach to this patient?

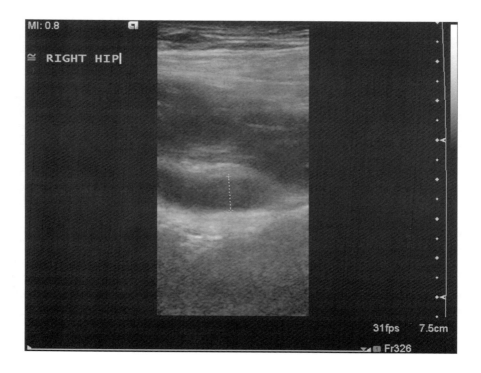

The casualty officer has sent some routine bloods and organized an ultrasound scan (USS) of his right hip which is shown above.

How would you assess the child and what is your management now based on the hip scan?

What is your approach to this patient?

I would want to assess the child to exclude an infectious cause for his symptoms such as a septic arthritis or osteomyelitis.

How would you assess the child and what is your management now based on the hip scan?

My clinical assessment would start with a detailed history from the parents.

On examination I would make an assessment of whether the child was well or unwell, and request a temperature measurement. I would assess the resting posture and range of motion of the hips. I may find the hip to be in a position of most comfort (flexed, abducted and externally rotated). I would also examine the whole lower limb, chest, abdomen, and spine.

The ultrasound shows an effusion around the hip which has been measured as 7 mm.

I would review the blood investigations taken.

I would organize AP and lateral radiographs of any affected part to rule out any underlying structural abnormality or fracture.

Four predictive markers of hip septic arthritis include:

1. Temperature > 38.5°C
2. White blood cells (WBC) > 12,000 cells/mm^3
3. ESR > 40
4. Non-weight bearing

The chance of there being a septic arthritis increases with the number of positive factors present [×1= 3%, ×2= 40% (treat as septic arthritis), ×3= 93%, /×4= 99.6%].

I would arrange an aspirate of the hip joint

If the aspirate revealed pus I would organize an open washout of the hip as soon as possible (urgent case < 6 h)

I would approach the hip through an anterior approach and remove an ellipse of capsule to allow free drainage after taking some deep tissue samples to send to microbiology and a copious washout with normal saline. I don't routinely use a hip spica post-operatively but recognize the risk of secondary subluxation and dysplasia that may develop in this condition. I would discuss appropriate antibiotics with the microbiologist, usually starting with broad spectrum and then adjusting, guided by the culture and sensitivities.

The child would require daily clinical and serial biochemical (inflammatory markers) review to make sure they improved. A prolonged course of antibiotics is advised. The child would also require longer-term follow-up to check the development and the growth of the hip joint.

Viva 16

You are asked to go and assess a newborn chid on the maternity ward.

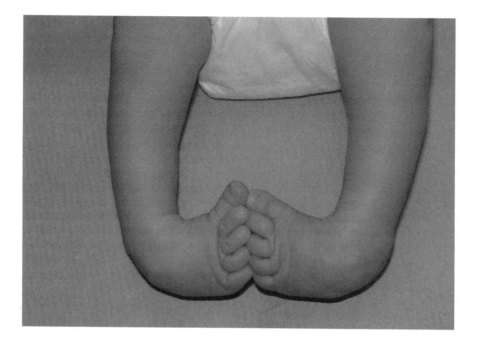

Describe the clinical photograph and the components of this deformity.

How do you classify the severity of this condition?

Describe the clinical photograph and the components of this deformity.

This is a clinical photograph of a newborn child with a clubfoot deformity (congenital talipes equino-varus). This is a complex three-dimensional deformity seen at birth with cavus and adductus of the midfoot and forefoot and varus and equinus of the hindfoot.

How do you classify the severity of this condition?

There are different scoring systems described to grade the severity of the deformity. In my institution we use the Pirani scoring system. It comprises two main scores, the midfoot contracture score and the hindfoot contracture score, which are combined to give a possible maximum total score of 6. (A high score correlates to a more deformed foot.) Each of these scores is made up of three separate components which are graded as 0, 0.5, or 1. The individual components of the deformity assessed are: severity of medial crease, coverage of the lateral head of talus, and curvature of the lateral border used in the midfoot score and rigidity of equinus, severity of the posterior crease, and degree of emptiness of heel for the hindfoot score.

How would you take your management from here?

I would manage this patient by taking a good history from the parents and examining the child to make sure they did not have any associated congenital anomalies or features which may suggest that this is a 'syndromic' club foot as opposed to an idiopathic clubfoot. I would then explain and start the Ponseti treatment programme, which is now recognized worldwide as an appropriate mainly non-operative approach to club foot treatment.

It starts with manipulation and serial casting.

The first key manoeuvre is to reduce the cavus deformity by dorsiflexing the first ray and unlocking the forefoot and midfoot. Elevation of the first ray produces supination so I warn the parents the foot may look worse after the first cast. The second important manoeuvre is to abduct the forefoot at midfoot level using the uncovered head of the talus laterally as a fulcrum.

Above-knee casts (with the knee at 90°) are applied with moulding into the corrected position and then each week the old cast is removed, the foot is scored and then subsequent casts are applied. The midfoot usually corrects well after four or five casts. If there is residual equinus (or less than 20° of dorsiflexion) of the hindfoot then this can be addressed by performing an Achilles tenotomy under a local or general anaesthetic. A final cast is applied for a further 3 weeks while the tenotomy heals.

Babies then go into Denis Browne boots with a bar (23 h a day for 3 months then just at night and naptime until the age of 5 years). This holds the affected foot externally rotated at about 70°. The vast majority of patients do very well and avoid the need for extensive surgical release. However, approximately 25% will require a tibialis anterior transfer laterally for residual deformity or inversion in swing after the age of about 4–5 years.

Viva 17

Here is a child with cerebral palsy.

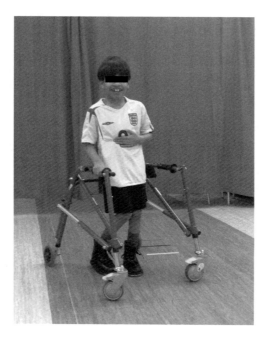

What is cerebral palsy and what different types do you know?

What is spasticity?

In what different ways do we manage spasticity?

Often ambulant children with cerebral palsy are assessed by gait analysis. What does that involve?

What is cerebral palsy and what different types do you know?

Cerebral palsy is a neuromuscular disorder caused by a non-progressive lesion to the immature developing brain (before the age of 2 years). Although the neurological injury is non-progressive, the musculoskeletal features evolve as the child grows.

Types of cerebral palsy are:

Anatomical—hemiplegia (40%)/diplegia (30%)/total body involvement (30%)

Physiological—spastic (60%)/dystonic (20%)/ataxic (10%)/hypotonic (10%)

Functional—classified by the Gross Motor Function Classification System (GMFCS)

What is spasticity?

Spasticity is the velocity-dependent increase in the tone of muscles (represents an increased response to stretch reflex).

In what different ways do we manage spasticity?

Principles include a multidisciplinary approach involving family and patient in goal planning, decisions about treatments, and exploring expectations.

Non-operative treatment is based around a physiotherapist who often acts as the main link between specialists. Adjuncts can be used to control spasticity including: botulinum toxin injections or baclofen (tablets or intrathecal pump).

- Botulinum toxin A (derived from *Clostridium botulinum*) is injected locally (dose is weight dependent) into spastic muscles. It works by preventing release of acetylcholine at the neuromuscular junction of those tight muscles and is effective for 3–6 months. It is often used in combination with plasters and targeted physiotherapy and/or orthotics to maintain an improved stretch
- Baclofen is a gamma-aminobutyric acid (GABA) agonist (an inhibitory neurotransmitter) which acts both centrally and peripherally to decrease spasticity. If administered intrathecally, via an infusion pump it allows an increased local dose with decreased systemic side-effects

Surgery is often needed, and appropriate planning and timing is crucial when performing multilevel surgery to avoid 'birthday syndrome'. Options can include bony surgery as well as soft tissue lengthening (without weakening) of tight muscles, as well as transfers of muscles to augment weak muscles.

Often ambulant children with cerebral palsy are assessed by gait analysis. What does that involve?

Gait analysis is the systematic description, assessment, and measurement of the quantities that characterize human locomotion. It involves the study of kinematics (the movements of the individual parts of the body) and kinetics (the forces and how they interact to produce those movements) as well as electromyography and energy consumption.

There is no defined standard; however, most gait laboratories will have two-dimensional video analysis and three-dimensional computer analysis, using specialized markers stuck onto specific bony landmarks. The computer program then breaks down the individual movements of anatomical parts into graphic form. Further detailed analysis involves the use of force plates, measuring ground reaction force, and electromyography, looking at muscle firing patterns.

It is important that the results of gait analysis are looked at in conjunction with a static detailed physical examination.

Viva 18

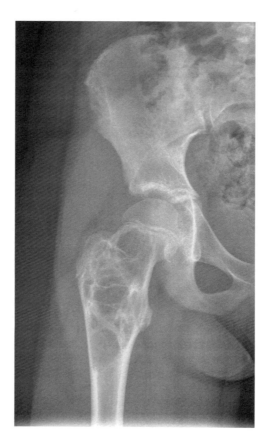

Can you describe this radiograph? What do you think the diagnosis is?

This patient presents with new-onset pain in the upper thigh. What do you think has happened?

How would you manage this patient now?

You treat expectantly, but unfortunately the lesion remains. How would you proceed now?

Can you describe the radiograph? What do you think the diagnosis is?

This is an AP radiograph showing a multiloculated lytic lesion in the proximal metaphysis of an immature individual. The zone of transition is sharp indicating this is likely to be a benign lesion with no associated periosteal reaction. Top of my diagnosis would be a loculated simple bone cyst, but an aneurysmal bone cyst is also a possibility.

This patient presents with new-onset pain in the upper thigh. What do you think has happened?

A lot of these lesions are found incidentally on radiographs taken for another reason, but new-onset pain in that area would suggest a pathological fracture through the weakened bone. A fallen fragment sign (cortex that has fallen into the cystic cavity) is pathognomonic of this.

How would you manage this patient now?

Having taken a thorough history and examined the patient, I would probably manage this expectantly as in a good percentage of patients the fracture actually stimulates new bone formation and with time the cyst fills in.

You treat expectantly but unfortunately the lesion remains. How would you proceed now?

If an expectant non-operative approach failed I would, under image guidance, aspirate the cyst and inject some steroid or bone graft/marrow to try and stimulate new bone formation. If this failed, a repeated attempt is worthwhile; however, the definitive surgical treatment would involve curetting out the lining of the cyst through a small cortical window and stabilizing the bone to prevent fracture. I would use flexible intramedullary nails across the lytic area. If the cavity is adjacent to the growth plate it is important not to damage it and risk growth arrest.

Viva 19

This 6-year-old child fell out of a tree onto their left arm.

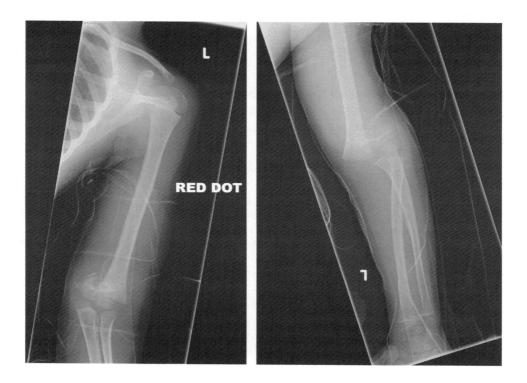

Can you describe the radiograph?

How would you manage this child?

You reduce and pin the fracture under anaesthetic, but on post-operative review in recovery you are unable to feel a pulse. What would you do now?

Can you describe the radiograph?

There is an 'off ended' Gartland 3 supracondylar fracture of the distal humerus.

How would you manage this child?

Assuming this was an isolated injury I would assess the child for the presence of an open injury, and also assess the distal neurovascular status (colour of hand, capillary refill of the fingertips, radial pulse, sensation in the specific dermatomes, and motor function of ulnar, radial, median, and anterior inter-osseus nerves).

I would organize for the child to have analgesia and a temporary backslab splint to stop the arm from moving and then mobilize my theatre team, as this child needs to go to theatre as soon as possible for closed reduction and percutaneous pinning.

In theatre, the set-up of the image intensifier and the help of a good assistant is key. The technique for reduction of these injuries is to apply good continuous traction (in 20° of flexion) for several minutes, then correct any valgus/varus and rotational deformity, before flexing up and hooking the distal fragment back on to the shaft. The forearm can be pronated to lock the fragments. I would insert a lateral wire first (1.6 mm), making sure I was through the far cortex. With that wire giving some stability, it is possible to extend the arm a little to plan a mini open approach to the medial side, allowing protection of the ulna nerve prior to inserting the cross wire. I would bend and cut the wires for ease of removal in the clinic in 3–4 weeks' time. I would splint the arm in a backslab in near extension. I would reassess the perfusion of the hand and watch for compartment syndrome.

You reduce and pin the fracture under anaesthetic, but on post-operative review in recovery you are unable to feel a pulse. What would you do now?

If I found no pulse in my post-operative review of the patient, I would make an assessment of the rest of the vascularity of the hand in terms of its colour and warmth and also the capillary refill time. If the hand was pink and warm with adequate capillary refill of the fingertips, then I would monitor the situation with regular review. The artery is likely to be in spasm and the pulse can take a day or two to recover. If the hand was white and capillary refill reduced, I would release the backslab and allow the arm to extend to see if this improved the situation. If not I would contact the vascular/plastic surgeons for an urgent review as the artery may have been caught up in the fracture and has now been occluded by the reduction. If so this would now require open exploration, usually via an anterior approach.

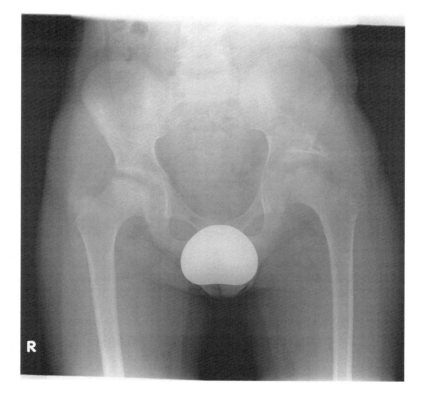

This radiograph shows a post-operative view of a boy's pelvis. What do you think the underlying diagnosis is and what procedure has he had?

What is the underlying disease and who gets it?

How do you classify this condition?

What are the principles of management?

This radiograph shows a post-operative view of a boy's pelvis. What do you think the underlying diagnosis is and what procedure has he had?

This is an AP pelvic radiograph of a skeletally immature patient showing flattening and deformity of both femoral heads in keeping with Perthes' disease. (Legg–Calve–Perthes disease). On the left side this patient has had a shelf procedure, which is a salvage type of acetabular procedure. It is an operation that redistributes the weight-bearing load of the femoral head through a larger surface area of pelvic cover.

What is the underlying disease and who gets it ?

Perthes' disease is idiopathic AVN of the proximal femoral epiphysis in childhood. It remains a controversial topic in orthopaedics because of its unknown aetiology and uncertain optimal treatment. It is more common in boys than girls by about 4:1 and it is bilateral in about 20% of cases.

How do you classify this condition?

There are many classifications used for Perthes' disease. Waldenström classified it into pathological stages:

1. Initial avascular event (crescent sign—representing a subchondral fracture)
2. Fragmentation (Herring's pillar classification)
3. Resolution—re-ossification
4. Remodelling—healed

The Herring classification of severity is based on the lateral pillar height on an AP radiograph during the fragmentation stage:

- B—more than 50% maintained
- C—less than 50% maintained

(A B/C border category was subsequently added.)

Catterall's classification contains four groups depending on the amount of femoral head involved on the lateral radiograph.

Catterall also added clinical and radiological 'head at risk signs' which he used to guide his management:

Clinical	Radiological
Obese	Horizontal physis
Progressive decreased ROM	Lateral subluxation of epiphysis
Abduction contracture	Lateral calcification
ER with flexion	Diffuse metaphyseal reaction
	Gage sign—inverted V-shaped lucency in lateral metaphysis

ROM, range of motion; ER, external rotation.

Stulberg's classification assessed the shape of femoral head at skeletal maturity and is used to predict who will do poorly in terms of early onset degenerative change:

I—normal
II—head spherical (magna/breva) and fits in socket which is congruent
III—mushroom head congruent
IV—flat head and flat socket congruent
V—flat head incongruent

What are the principles of management?

Goals of treatment are:

1. Symptomatic relief
2. Containment of the head and hence correct development
3. Restoration of ROM

These goals can be achieved by various non-operative and operative treatments which still are debated around the world.

Each patient should be managed on an individual basis taking into account their age, clinical signs, and radiological appearances on X-ray.

Viva Table 2

Basic Sciences

Section 3 Tissue Anatomy and Pathology

Viva 21

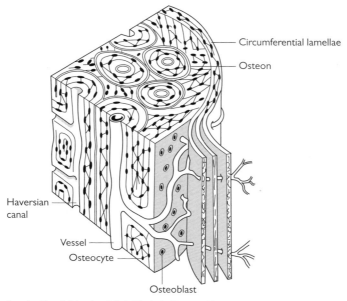

Circumferential lamellae

Osteon

Haversian canal

Vessel

Osteocyte

Osteoblast

What is bone?

How do osteoblasts and osteoclasts differ?

What is Wolff's law?

What is bone?

Bone is a composite dynamic form of specialized connective tissue.

It comprises cells (10%) and extracellular matrix (90%).

The cells include osteoblasts, osteocytes, and osteoclasts.

The matrix has organic (collagens, mainly type 1) and inorganic (calcium phosphate, osteocalcium phosphate) constituents.

Bone functions to move, support, and protect the internal organs, it produces red and white blood cells, and contains the majority of calcium and phosphate in the body.

How do osteoblasts and osteoclasts differ?

Osteoblasts are derived from undifferentiated mesenchymal cells; they are bone forming and lay down osteoid (type 1 collagen) as well as activating osteoclasts to resorb bone via the receptor activator of nuclear factor kappa-B (RANK) ligand (RANKL) system. These processes are controlled by cytokines, growth factors and bone morphogenic protein (BMP).

Osteoclasts are from a haemopoietic monocyte cell lineage. They are multinucleated giant cells that resorb bone. They can sit in small pits called Howships lacunae, on the bone surface, or lead cutting cones that tunnel through the bone. Under their ruffled brush border, with an increased surface area, they create a low-pH microenvironment which dissolves the inorganic apatite crystals. Enzymes are released (tartrate resistant acid phosphatase, TRAP) and proteases then break down the organic matrix components. This process is controlled via the RANKL system (inhibited by osteoprotegrin) of activated osteoblasts.

Osteocytes are osteoblasts that have become trapped in bone matrix (making up to 90% of the cells in bone), they have an important role in homeostasis of calcium and phosphate metabolism.

What is Wolff's law?

Wolff's law is a theory developed by the German anatomist/surgeon Julius Wolff in the 19th century. It states that bone will adapt to the loads placed through or across it. It is the result of the close coupling within bone remodelling units consisting of osteoblast, osteoclast, and supporting stromal tissues. If loading on a particular bone increases, the bone will remodel itself over time to become stronger to resist that sort of loading.

In relation to soft tissue, Davis's law explains how soft tissue remoulds itself according to imposed demands.

Viva 22

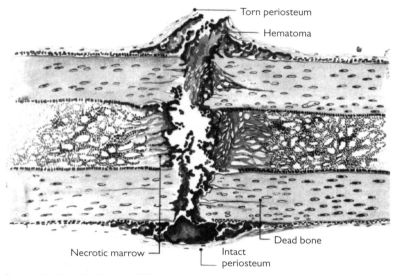

Torn periosteum
Hematoma
Dead bone
Necrotic marrow
Intact periosteum

Tell me how bones unite after a fracture.

What is the difference between intramembranous and endochondral ossification?

How do bones get wider?

Tell me how bones unite after a fracture.

Secondary fracture healing can be divided into five stages: haematoma; inflammatory reaction; soft callus formation; hard callus formation and remodelling; however, in reality these stages merge into a continuum.

Haematoma (hours)

The damaged tissue surfaces and blood vessels results in vasoconstriction and haematoma formation—platelet plugs form and the activated platelets degranulate releasing platelet-derived growth factor (PDGF). The clotting cascade and the complement system are both activated—these are step-wise amplification cascades that result in the activation of cytokines and signalling molecules which are chemotactic to the inflammatory cells and angiogenic to blood vessels. Released opsonins attach to bacteria and dead necrotic cells to expedite their phagocytosis. BMPs (BMP 7 is important) are also released from damaged bone straight away; they are osteoinductive, mitogenic, and angiogenic.

Inflammatory phase (days)

The arrival and activation of polymorph neutrophils (which also release activated cytokines and leukotrienes) is the start of the inflammatory phase. A bit later the next cells to arrive are the macrophages which start to phagocytose dead cells and tissue.

Angiogenesis has started and helps to bring in new undifferentiated mesenchymal cells.

Repair phase—soft to hard callus (weeks)

The end of the inflammatory phase occurs with the arrival of fibroblasts and the beginning of the repair phase.

This phase can be thought of with regard to:

1. The mechanical environment which delineates which cells form from the undifferentiated mesenchymal cells
2. The biochemical environment (oxygen tension and pH (haematoma is acidic—osteoblasts need an alkaline environment to lay down bone)

A fracture gap strain of 200% promotes fibroblast proliferation—fibrous tissue forms in the fracture gap and it becomes less mobile (angiogenesis continues). Less than 15% strain and chondrocytes proliferate laying down collagen matrix and soft callus in the fracture gap. With 2–5% strain the osteoblasts start to lay down osteoid which is then mineralized to form hard callus (woven bone).

Remodelling phase (months to years)

The last phase, which lasts many months, is remodelling where disorganized woven bone is stress orientated into hard dense lamellar bone (obeying the mechanical principles of Wolff's law).

What is the difference between intramembranous and endochondral ossification?

Endochondral ossification is the process associated with foetal bone development, day-to-day bone growth, and to a certain extent fracture repair. The replacement of cartilage by bone is called endochondral ossification. This is the type of bone formation found in the development of long bones such as the femur and humerus.

Intramembranous ossification is the formation of bone on, or in, fibrous connective tissue (which is formed from condensed mesenchyme cells). Intramembraneous ossification is the process used to make flat bones such as the mandible and flat bones of the skull.

How do bones get wider?

The increase in diameter is called appositional growth. Osteoblasts in the periosteum form compact bone around the external bone surface. At the same time, osteoclasts in the endosteum break down bone on the internal bone surface, around the medullary cavity. These two processes together increase the diameter of the bone.

Viva 23

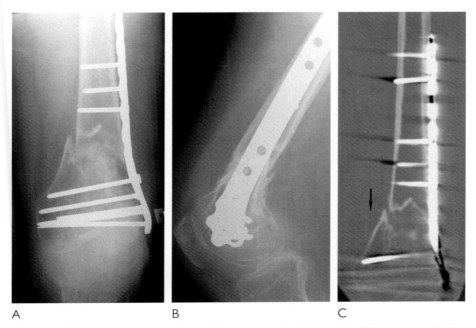

A   B   C

This patient fractured a femur 4 months ago, but is still getting significant pain. What do you see and how would you manage it?

What factors influence fracture healing?

This patient fractured a femur 4 months ago, but is still getting significant pain; what do you see and how would you manage it?

This is an AP radiograph showing a supracondylar fracture treated with a locking plate device. The fracture doesn't show any signs of healing and at 4 months' post-fixation this would be an established non-union.

First infection must be excluded as this can also cause non-union.

If not infected:

- Open debridement
- Bone graft (iliac crest graft)
- Additional BMPs?
- Fixation—repeat internal or external (Ilizarov)

What factors influence fracture healing?

1. Fracture mechanical environment
2. Local biology
   Blood supply
   Degree of soft tissue injury
   Open or closed injury
   Degree of fragmentation/bone loss
   Site of fracture (metaphyseal versus diaphyseal)
   Soft tissue interposition
   Stability (cf. absolute/relative/dynamization)
   Presence of infection
   Presence of pathological lesion
   Previous irradiation to that area
3. Systemic biology
   Age
   Smoking
   Drugs—non-steroidal anti-inflammatory drugs (NSAIDs), steroids, bisphosphonates
   Medical co-morbidities—diabetes mellitus (DM)
   Nutrition
   Associated head injury

Viva 24

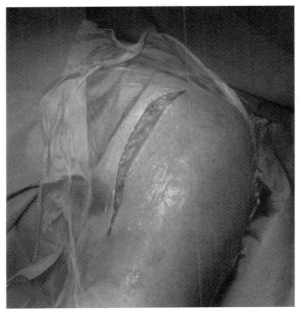

Can you describe the deltopectoral approach to the glenohumeral joint?

Can you describe the patient set-up, primary, and secondary portals for ankle arthroscopy?

Can you describe the deltopectoral approach to the glenohumeral joint?

NB: You should be able do the same thing for all common approaches.

General anaesthetic ± interscalene block.

Beach chair position.

Incision is from 1–2 cm inferior to the tip of the coracoid process extending towards the anterior axillary fold. The deltopectoral groove is identified by a 'yellow stripe' of fat and the cephalic vein is sought lying in the groove. The vein is usually reflected laterally. The interval between the deltoid and the pectoralis major is developed and the conjoined tendon arising from the coracoid process is identified. The conjoined tendon is now dissected free from the underlying subscapularis. The conjoined tendon is retracted medially with the help of the self-retaining retractors (± partial division 1 cm distal to the coracoid). The subscapularis muscle and its tendon are identified by externally rotating the arm. Stay sutures are used to control the medial musculotendinous tissues of the subscapularis. With the arm in ER, division of the subscapularis tendon is carried out about 1–2 cm from its insertion just lateral to the musculotendinous junction. Depending on indication, the subscapularis muscle is then either stripped off the anterior capsule or the capsule is divided with the tendon.

Nerves at risk

- The axillary nerve lies just inferior to the shoulder joint capsule. A blunt ring-handled retractor is slipped down on the anterior capsule and passed inferior to the shoulder, retracting the inferior structures including the axillary nerve away from the capsule, thereby protecting this important nerve which lies only 5–10 mm below the inferior capsular fold
- The musculocutaneous nerve

Can you describe the patient set-up, primary, and secondary portals for ankle arthroscopy?

Ankle portals

1. Anteromedial: initial arthroscopy is performed with the scope in the anteromedial portal, but for the majority of cases this portal will be used for instrumentation, located at the level of the ankle joint, just medial to the tibialis anterior tendon, and located about 5 mm lateral to the medial malleolus. An 18-gauge syringe is used to infuse saline into the joint; the greater saphenous nerve and vein are at risk with this portal, lying 7–9 mm medial to the portal

2. Anterolateral: once the joint is distended with saline, use an 18-gauge needle to mark the location of the anterolateral portal which should lie just lateral to the peroneus tertius tendon; staying lateral to the peroneus tertius, helps avoid injury to the dorsal lateral branch of the peroneal nerve. Use the scope to transilluminate the anterolateral skin, in order to look for underlying cutaneous nerves; the scope can then be driven forward (elevating the synovium and skin) which further assists with placement of this portal. Make a small incision and then spread with a hemostat; be aware that the intermediate branch of the superficial peroneal nerve is about 5–6 mm from this portal

NB: You should be able to do the same thing for the knee and the shoulder.

Viva 25

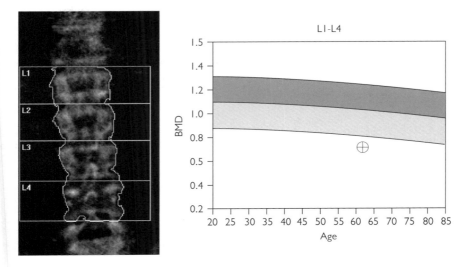

Results Summary:

Region	Area[cm²]	BMC[(g)]	BMD[(g/cm²)]	T-score	PR (Peak Reference)	Z-score	AM (Age Matched)
LI	17.25	13.34	0.773	−2.7	72	−2.1	77
L2	17.89	12.60	0.746	−3.2	68	−2.5	73
L3	17.72	12.64	0.713	−3.5	65	−2.9	69
L4	18.84	11.87	0.630	−4.2	58	−3.5	62
Total	70.70	50.45	0.714	−3.4	65	−2.8	70

Reproduced from Raashid Luqmani, Theodore Pincus, and Maarten Boers, *Rheumatoid Arthritis* (Oxford Rheumatology Library), 2010, Figure 8.2, p. 84, with permission from Oxford University Press. .

What investigation is illustrated above?

Define osteoporosis and list its risk factors.

What numerical results are given by this test and how do you interpret them?

Can you describe the treatment of osteoporosis, the drugs, and how they act?

What investigation is illustrated above?

A bone-density scan.

Define osteoporosis and list its risk factors.

Osteoporosis is a condition in which decreased bone mineral density results in increased susceptibility to low-trauma fragility fractures.

Osteoporosis (in women) is defined by the World Health Organization as a bone mineral density 2.5 standard deviations below peak bone mass (20-year-old healthy female average) as measured on a dual-energy X-ray absorptiometry (DEXA) scan.

Risk factors for osteoporosis include:

- Low-impact fracture
- New thoracic kyphosis
- Early menopause < 48 years [oestrogen blocks the effect of parathyroid hormone (PTH) on osteoclasts]
- Family history of hip or vertebral fracture in first-degree relative < 65 years old
- Predisposing pathology: hypothyroid, rheumatoid arthritis (RA), alcohol, Cushing's, malignancy
- Prolonged amenorrhoea in the absence of pregnancy
- Drugs: steroids, thyroxine, heparin, phenytoin, chemotherapy

What numerical results are given by this test and how do you interpret them?

Really, there are only four important numbers, and two of these are of lesser importance:

1. First, identify the percentage of normal bone density for the patient's age. This is helpful in your explanation to patients, but doesn't really affect diagnosis or treatment. (This is one of the numbers you can ignore if you wish)
2. Second, find the Z-score, which is the standard deviation (SD) from normal for that patient's age group. (This is the other number you can ignore)
3. Third, find the percentage of bone density compared with normal young adults. This number has a powerful impact on patients. Ninety per cent and above is considered normal. It is important to tell patients that this is the amount of bone that they *have* compared to what they *had* or *should have had* at the age of 40
4. Fourth, find the T-score, which is the number of standard deviations from normal young adults. *This is the key number* as it is from this that the World Health Organization takes its *definition of osteoporosis*. The T-score shows where your patient is compared with the population. In other words, an Irish woman with a small frame stacks up differently from an African American woman with a larger frame, and you want to know how they compare with people of their own sex, race, age, height, and weight. The T-score predicts fracture risk: For every −1 SD the fracture risk doubles. Osteoporosis is defined as a T-score > 2.5 SD below mean (lumbar spine) [the bone mineral density (BMD) of a fit and healthy 25-year-old]

Can you describe the treatment of osteoporosis, the drugs, and how they act?

Treatment guidelines from the National Institute of Health and Clinical Excellence (NICE) are divided into lifestyle changes and pharmacological treatment.

All at-risk patients and those with confirmed osteoporosis (either by fracture or DEXA scan) should have information regarding lifestyle changes which include taking weight-bearing exercise, reducing alcohol consumption, stopping smoking, and reducing falls risk.

All patients should have calcium (1500 mg) and vitamin D (800 IU) supplements.

Female patients who are post-menopausal < 65 years old with T-score > 3 or > 75 years old with osteoporotic fracture should have:

- First-line treatment—bisphosphonates. Alendronate 70 mg once a week
- Second-line treatment—strontium ranelate 2 mg once daily (may affect future DEXA scans)
- Third-line treatment—raloxifene 60 mg once daily

Bisphosphonates are the main pharmacological measures for treatment. They work by inhibiting osteoclast function and hence resorption of bone. They attach to the osteoclast and prevent the attachment of its ruffled brush border to the bone.

Strontium ranelate stimulates proliferation of the osteoblasts, as well as inhibiting the proliferation of osteoclasts.

Raloxifene is a selective oestrogen receptor modulator. It works by attaching itself to oestrogen receptors in the bone, stimulating the production of new bone.

Three key elements of a strategy for osteoporotic fractures are:

1. High-quality fracture care—delivered through coordinated multidisciplinary teamwork
2. High-quality secondary prevention of fragility fracture—ensured by providing bone protection and falls assessment
3. High-quality information—using standards, audit and feedback to improve hip fracture care and secondary prevention

Note: osteopenia = T-score–2.5 to–1.0. Treat with lifestyle changes only.

Viva 26

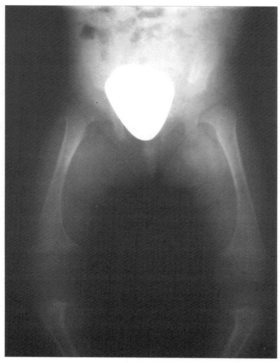

The radiograph above was performed on a child who presented with bowed legs.

What do you think the diagnosis is?

What is rickets?

What are the causes of rickets?

How else might a child with rickets present, and how would you investigate them?

What do you think the diagnosis is?

This plain radiograph of the pelvis and knees shows generalized widening of the metaphysis and cupping of the epiphysis in keeping with a metabolic condition such as rickets. Differential diagnosis would include a generalized skeletal dysplasia.

What is rickets?

Rickets is a disease of growing bone that is unique to children and adolescents. It is caused by a failure of osteoid to calcify in a growing person. Failure of osteoid to calcify in adults is called osteomalacia.

What are the causes of rickets?

- Nutritional rickets. (There are few dietary sources of vitamin D. The best ones are fatty fish such as salmon and sardines, and margarines supplemented with vitamin D. Milk contains added vitamin D in the USA but not in the UK. Most people in the UK get most of their vitamin D from exposure of the skin to sunlight)
- Lack of sunlight
- Congenital rickets
- Rickets of prematurity
- Vitamin D resistance (type I and type II)
- Neoplastic rickets
- Hypophosphataemic rickets
- Drug-induced rickets

How else might a child with rickets present, and how would you investigate them?

The child may present with generalized muscular hypotonia of an unknown mechanism. In the long bones, laying down of uncalcified osteoid at the metaphyses leads to spreading of those areas, producing knobby deformity which is visualized on radiography as cupping and flaring of the metaphyses. Weight bearing produces deformities such as bowlegs and knock-knees. In the chest, knobbly deformities results in the rachitic rosary along the costochondral junctions. The weakened ribs pulled by muscles also produce flaring over the diaphragm, which is known as the Harrison groove. The sternum may be pulled into a pigeon-breast deformity. At the ankle, palpation of the tibial malleolus gives the impression of a double epiphysis (Marfan sign).

Blood tests

Early on in the disease course, the calcium (ionized fraction) is low; however, it is often within the reference range at the time of diagnosis as PTH levels increase. Calcidiol (25-hydroxy vitamin D) levels are low, and PTH levels are elevated; however, determining calcidiol and PTH levels is typically not necessary. Alkaline phosphatase levels are elevated.

Viva 27

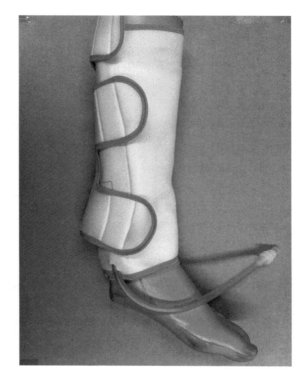

Do you use this device in your clinical practice?

Describe Virchow's triad and the risk factors for formation of a deep vein thrombosis (DVT).

What risk levels do you quote to patients undergoing total hip replacement (THR) and total knee replacement (TKR)?

What is your DVT prophylaxis policy for THR in a 70-year-old man with no significant additional risk factors?

Do you use this device in your clinical practice?

Yes, this is a mechanical calf pump that we use intra-operatively to prevent venous thrombosis.

Describe Virchow's triad and the risk factors for formation of a deep vein thrombosis (DVT).

Virchow's triad includes:

1. Hypercoagulable state
2. Stasis of vascular flow
3. Damage to the vascular endothelium

What risk levels do you quote to patients undergoing total hip replacement (THR) and total knee replacement (TKR)?

Forty to 60 per cent of THR patients who do not receive prophylaxis will get a DVT (dependent on imaging method). With chemical and mechanical prophylaxis asymptomatic DVT occurs in 10% of THR and 20% of TKR patients. Symptomatic DVT occurs in 1.3% of TKR patients and 2.81% of THR patients.

What is your DVT prophylaxis policy for THR in a 70-year-old man with no significant additional risk factors?

The two main strategies for prevention are:

1. Non-pharmacological interventions. These include anti-DVT stockings and foot or calf pumps
2. Pharmacological interventions. These include one or more of the following:
   - Low-molecular-weight heparin (LMWH): heparin and LMWH are equivalent in preventing DVT, although LMWH has greater bioavailability, longer duration of anticoagulant effect in fixed doses, and little requirement for laboratory monitoring, and is thus more cost-effective
   - Fondaparinux sodium (Arixtra)—a synthetic pentasaccharide. When used at 2.5 mg subcutaneously (SC) four times a day post-operatively, it significantly improves the risk-to-benefit ratio for the prevention of post-operative venous thromboembolism
   - Warfarin—an effective but cumbersome DVT prophylaxis regimen is achieved with either a fixed or an adjusted dose
   - Aspirin—however, there is not much evidence of its efficacy

You should be able to quote your local policy on what they use in this situation.

Viva Table 2

Basic Sciences

Section 4 Mechanics and Tribology

Viva 28

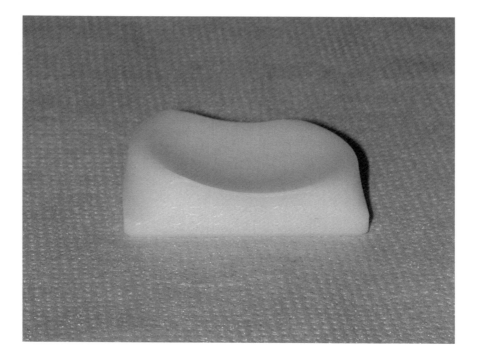

What is this material?

How is it manufactured?

How can its material properties be manipulated?

What is this material?

This is an ultra-high-molecular-weight polyethylene (UHMWPE) component from a unicompartmental knee replacement. UHMWPE is a long hydrocarbon chain held together by covalent bonds. The chain exists in two phases; a disorganized amorphous phase and a more organized crystalline phase. Three types are available (GUR 1020, 1050, 1090) which have increasing molecular weight.

How is it manufactured?

It is manufactured using the Zeigler process as follows:

1. Ethylene gas is polymerized in a low-temperature, low-pressure environment. The catalyst used is titanium chloride. This produces a fine UHMWPE powder
2. The UHMWPE powder is then processed by one of the following methods:
   Ram extrusion: produces bar stock, lowest quality
   Sheet compression moulding: higher quality
   Direct compression moulding (e.g. Arcom by Biomet): the UHMWPE powder is moulded into the shape of the final component. Better quality control, but expensive
3. Machining: UHMWPE bar, sheets, or moulded components are shaped into their final form
4. Sterilization and packaging: by gamma irradiation, gas plasma, or ethylene oxide

How can its material properties be manipulated?

By making cross-linked polyethylene (XLPE).

The manufacture of XLPE involves bombarding the material with an electron beam or gamma irradiation, which causes chain scission of double covalent bonds, followed by rebonding, either by oxidation or cross-linking between adjacent polymer chains. To prevent oxidation due to the formation of free radicals, the process is performed in an inert environment (a vacuum or noble gas). XLPE must be annealed, to release oxygen free radicals from the material, as they will cause slow oxidation and therefore reduce shelf life.Some manufacturers add antioxidants (e.g. vitamin E).

* Advantages of XLPE are: 80–100% reduction of *in vivo* wear
* Disadvantages of XLPE are: it is more brittle and therefore at increased risk of fracture (there is debate as to whether it is suitable for use in the knee)

Viva 29

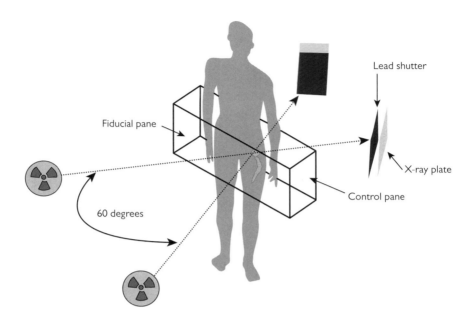

What is shown in this picture?

How does it work?

What is it used for?

What is shown in this picture?

A Roentgen stereophotogrammetric analysis (RSA).

How does it work?

RSA is a method for determining the three-dimensional coordinates of an object within the calibration cage, from two two-dimensional X-ray images. Tantalum marker beads are inserted into bone at the time of surgery. Post-operatively, the subject is placed within the calibration cage, which contains tantalum marker beads placed at accurately measured points. Two X-ray sources are placed at a known angle to each other. Stereo X-ray images are then taken simultaneously. The distance between the X-ray sources and the calibration cage is known; therefore the three-dimensional coordinates of any point on the two-dimensional stereo X-ray images can be determined.

What is it used for?

RSA is predominantly used to measure the 'migration', over time, of joint replacements. It is used as a surrogate measure of outcome and has been shown to be an accurate predictor of failure in total hip arthroplasty. Most joint replacements migrate during the first 2 years of implantation. If there is rapid, sustained migration during this period, then there is an increased risk of failure. RSA is therefore a useful tool for evaluating new designs of joint replacement. It is a powerful technique, which means that only about 20 patients are required per study, which typically takes 2 years to complete. The direction of migration is important and is design-dependent. For example, when an Exeter stem has 1.5 mm of distal migration, this is not associated with an increased risk of failure. Conversely, a distal migration of 1.5 mm in the Charnley-Elite stem is associated with a 30% failure rate at 8 years.

Viva 30

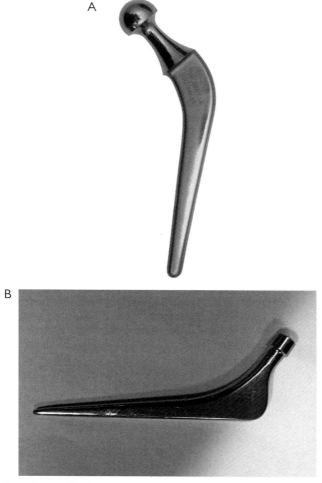

A

B

Photograph courtesy of Paul Cooper.

What are these devices?

What are the characteristic features of these designs?

Tell me about their design philosophy? How do they work?

How do they fail?

What are these devices?

These are two cemented stems. The first is an evolution of the Charnley stem; the second is the Exeter stem.

What are the characteristic features of these designs?

The Charnley-type stem is an example of a composite beam design, which has a collar or flange and a rough surface finish.

The Exeter is an example of a polished, double-tapered stem.

Tell me about their design philosophy? How do they work?

The composite beam or 'shape-closed' design philosophy relies on friction to maintain the position of the stem within the cement mantle. A rough surface finish (typically greater than 2 Ra) and design features, such as a collar or flange are intended to minimize micromotion at the prosthesis–cement interface. The Exeter stem works on the taper slip (or force-closed) principle, whereby stability is achieved by allowing micromovement at the prosthesis–cement interface. These devices have design features that promote migration, these include a collarless geometry and a highly polished surface finish (<0.01 Ra). Polished, tapered stems subside within the cement mantle, and in so doing they generate radial stresses which increase compression at the bone–cement and prosthesis–cement interfaces. In turn, this stabilizes the bone–cement–prosthesis composite. The viscoelastic properties of cement (creep and stress relaxation) are a key factor in this process.

How do they fail?

Composite beam stems fail when movement occurs at the prosthesis–cement interface. A rough surface finish will abrade the cement mantle once micromovement is established. This probably leads to gap formation, which in turn further increases micromovement and also allows the circulation of wear debris. Polished, tapered stems are inherently stable devices and their mechanism of failure is not well understood. RSA and retrieval studies suggest that these devices fail when they rotate in the axial plane.

Viva 31

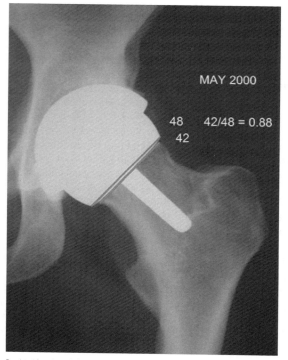

MAY 2000

48   42/48 = 0.88
42

Reprinted from Journal of Arthroplasty, 23, 8, Spencer, S., Carter, R., Murray, H., and Meek, R.M., 'Femoral neck narrowing after metal-on-metal hip resurfacing', pp. 1105–1109, Copyright 2008, with permission from Elsevier..

What type of bearing is this?

What are its advantages over a conventional bearing surface?

What factors influence the type of lubrication achieved?

Are there any adverse effects with this type of bearing?

What type of bearing is this?

This is a hip resurfacing arthroplasty, with a large-diameter, cobalt–chrome, metal-on-metal bearing.

What are its advantages over a conventional bearing surface?

1. Low wear: after an initial period of bedding-in wear, these devices have a linear wear rate of less than 0.01 mm/year, compared with metal on UHMWPE bearings which have a linear wear rate of 0.1–0.2 mm/year
2. Hydrodynamic lubrication: hip simulator studies suggest that a large-head metal-on-metal articulation is capable of fluid-film lubrication. It is likely that boundary lubrication occurs when the hip is at rest and a fluid film only when the hip is moving

What factors influence the type of lubrication achieved?

1. Radial clearance: this is the gap between the acetabular and femoral bearing surfaces. A large radial clearance results in polar bearing and boundary lubrication. A small radial clearance may result in equatorial bearing. There is therefore an optimal radial clearance for each size of femoral component, which is small enough to allow fluid-film lubrication but large enough to prevent excessive wear and cold-welding
2. Femoral head diameter: large femoral heads are more likely to induce fluid-film lubrication
3. Component position: a high cup abduction angle can increase the risk of edge loading which in turn results in boundary lubrication

Are there any adverse effects with this type of bearing?

1. Cancer risk: metal-on-metal articulations produces large numbers of very small wear particles. In addition, high levels of cobalt and chrome are measured in the blood of patients with this type of bearing surface. There is concern, although no definitive evidence, that this may increase the risk of developing some types of cancer
2. Inflammatory masses: some patients with metal-on-metal hip resurfacing arthroplasty have developed large, local inflammatory masses caused by metal wear debris

Viva 32

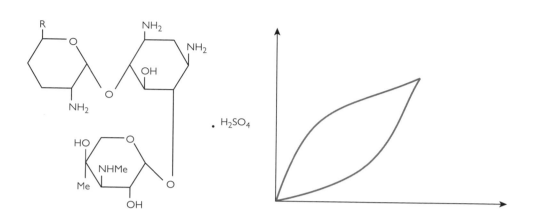

. H_2SO_4

This is the chemical structure of a material we commonly use in joint arthroplasty—what do you think it is?

What is it made of?

What happens when the powder and liquid are mixed?

What are its material properties?

What factors influence its properties?

This is the chemical structure of a material we commonly use in joint arthroplasty—what do you think it is?

Bone cement.

What is it made of?

The main components are powder and liquid:

1. Powder:
   - Pre-polymerized poly methyl methacrylate (PMMA)
   - Barium sulphate
2. Liquid:
   - Mono methyl methacrylate (MMA, monomer)
   - N-dimethyl-p-toluidine, which acts as an accelerator
   - Hydroquinone, which acts as an inhibitor
   - Colour, e.g. chlorophyll

What happens when the powder and liquid are mixed?

Solid cement is formed through an exothermic free-radical polymerization reaction. It occurs in two phases. During the first phase polymer chains form, resulting in shrinkage of the material. During the second phase of polymerization, the temperature rises and the cement undergoes thermal expansion.

What are its material properties?

Cement is a viscoelastic material and has the following properties:

1. Creep: increasing strain under a constant load (stress)
2. Stress relaxation: a reduction in stress under a constant strain
3. Hysteresis: refers to the process by which a viscoelastic substance loses energy when a load is applied, then removed

What factors influence its properties?

1. Porosity—vacuum mixing improves fatigue strength
2. Antibiotics

Viva 33

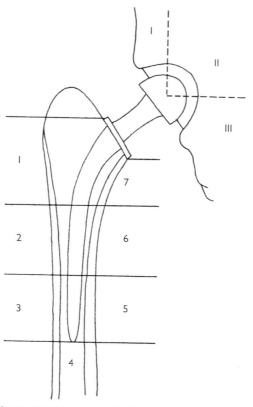

Reproduced from C. Bulstrode et al., Oxford Textbook of Trauma and Orthopaedics second edition, 2011, figure 7.10.3, p. 586, with permission from Oxford University Press..

What does this diagram represent?

What is the pathological process behind aseptic loosening?

What does this diagram represent?

The diagram shows the potential areas of lucency around the femoral and acetabular components of a total hip replacement according to Gruen (femur) and DeLee and Charnley (cup).

What is the pathological process behind aseptic loosening?

Osteolysis in total joint replacement is thought to occur as a result of resorption of bone by osteo-clasts at the bone–cement interface and is associated with aseptic implant loosening. Polyethylene wear debris produced at the bearing surfaces combined with cement debris formed from movement at the interfaces is thought to induce osteolysis. *In vitro* studies suggest that the activated macrophage is a key intermediary in this process.

Peri-prosthetic bone resorption involves a series of complicated interactions between macrophages and osteoclasts. Osteolysis occurs due to both the direct resorption of bone, as a consequence of osteoclast stimulation and, to a lesser extent, the secretion of enzymes from other cells (such as met-alloproteinases from fibroblasts). Macrophages are thought to be pivotal in the osteolysis process.

Cell culture studies have demonstrated that particulate wear debris from prosthetic materials are *phagocytosed* by macrophages, which subsequently respond in one of two ways:

- Firstly they secrete numerous cellular mediators some of which [tumour necrosis factor-alpha (TNF-α), interleukin (IL)-6, IL-1, and prostaglandin 2 (PGE2)] are able to induce cell proliferation and bone resorption in osteoclasts
- Secondly, *in vitro* studies have demonstrated that activated macrophages are able to differentiate into osteoclasts via two distinct pathways (fibroblast RANKL activated and TNF-α activated)

Viva 34

This is a stress–strain curve for a generic material.

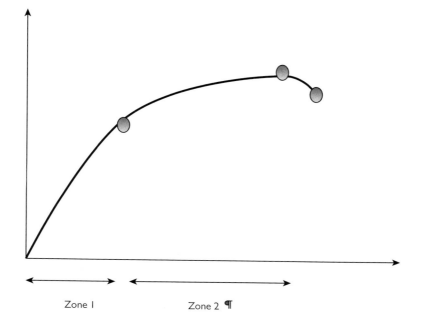

Zone 1

Zone 2 ¶

What does Zone 1 represent?

What is Young's modulus?

What does the first circle represent?

What is Zone 2?

What do the second and third circles represent?

What is strain hardening?

What does Zone 1 represent?

The elastic zone: a material is perfectly elastic if the strain reduces to zero when the stress is removed.

What is Young's modulus?

Young's modulus is stress/strain in the elastic region and is a measure of the stiffness of the material. (The higher the Young's modulus, i.e. steeper the slope, the higher the stiffness.)

What does the first circle represent?

It represents the proportional limit, which is the point at which the zone of elasticity ends. At this point, a sudden elongation of the material occurs without a significant increase in the applied load.

What is Zone 2?

The plastic zone: during this phase the material will not regain its original length when the load is removed.

What do the second and third circles represent?

The second circle is the point of ultimate strength; this is the point of maximum stress. The stress gradually reduces as the strain increases and the material fails at the third circle. The area under the curve represents the 'energy to failure'.

What is strain hardening?

Strain hardening is the increase in stress upon yield stress.

Viva 35

This is a screw from a basic small fragment set used in fracture fixation.

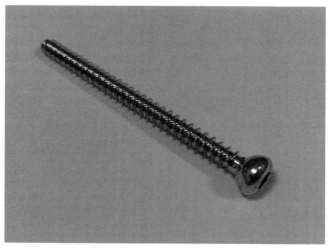

Picture courtesy of Synthes UK Ltd. .

Can you take me through the different parts of the screw and their function?

What mechanical properties does a screw have?

How does the small fragment screw differ mechanically from this locking bolt for an intramedullary nail?

What size drills would you use to insert the small fragment screw to act as a lag screw across a fracture?

Can you take me through the different parts of the screw and their function?

Head—provides attachment for a screwdriver (hexagonal for six points of contact to increase torque, avoid slip, and improve directional control).

Counter-sink.

Run out—transitional area between head and thread (relatively weak area).

Shaft—inner core diameter (tensile strength proportional to radius cubed).

Thread—outer diameter (proportional to pull out strength), partially threaded versus fully threaded (80% grip of near cortex and 20% grip of far cortex).

Crest/root of the thread.

Pitch (lead)—distance advanced for one 360° turn (cancellous > cortical > locking).

Flutes—removes swarf (bone debris).

Tip—difference between cortical (blunt) and cancellous screw (corkscrew).

What mechanical properties does a screw have?

A screw is a device that converts a torsional force into a linear force.

The effective thread depth is a combination of pitch and thread (outer diameter) which is proportional to pull-out strength.

The tensile strength is proportional to the inner core radius cubed.

How does the small fragment screw differ mechanically from this locking bolt for an intramedullary nail?

A locking bolt is there to create a rotationally stable construct. It has a wide inner core diameter (ultimate tensile stress, UTS) relative to a small thread (it doesn't need a large amount of pull-out strength).

What size drills would you use to insert the small fragment screw to act as a lag screw across this fracture?

Large lag hole (near cortex) = 3.5 mm drill.

Small hole (far cortex) 2.5 mm.

Viva Table 2

Basic Sciences

Section 5 Statistics and Orthopaedic Imaging

Viva 36

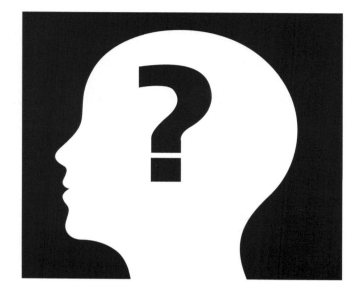

What is a hypothesis?

What is a null hypothesis?

How would you go about setting up a clinical trial?

What are Type 1 and Type 2 errors?

What is a hypothesis?

A hypothesis is a proposition that serves as a starting point for further investigation.

What is a null hypothesis?

A null hypothesis is a primary assumption that any differences between different groups seen in your study occurred purely by chance.

How would you go about setting up a clinical trial?

1. Identify a problem/interest to be studied—via literature search—and identify a gold standard to compare with
2. Ask a scientific question—define a null hypothesis to test
3. Design your study:
   - Define your population—inclusion / exclusion criteria
   - Methodology of study—randomized/double blinded (masked)/stratification for confounding factors
   - Power analysis (statistician) for numbers required to able to draw statistically valid conclusions from your results
   - Define outcome measures (valid and reproducible)
4. Obtain ethics approval from local or national committee
5. Register trial
6. Conduct the trial
7. Recruit your patients—collect your data
8. Analyse your results (stats)
9. Interpret your findings, write up your work, and publish in peer-reviewed journals

What are Type 1 and Type 2 errors?

A Type 1 or alpha error occurs when a researcher's false hypothesis is accepted—in other words a null hypothesis that is true is falsely rejected or the p-value suggests there is significant difference when there isn't. It is protected against by having high levels of significance. The level that is usually selected for biological studies is 95%.

A Type 2 or beta error occurs when a researcher's hypothesis that is true cannot be demonstrated—in other words a null hypothesis is falsely accepted or the p-value suggests there is no difference when there is. This is protected against by increasing the power of the study, i.e. increasing the numbers being analysed.

Viva 37

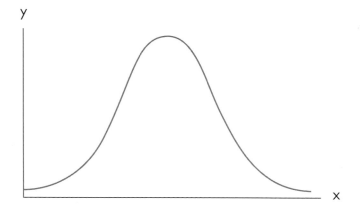

What kinds of data are there in orthopaedic surgical literature and what common statistical tests are used for these data?

What do you understand by the sensitivity and specificity of a test?

What factors do you look for in an outcome scoring system?

What kinds of data are there in orthopaedic surgical literature and what common statistical tests are used for these data?

There are discrete data which are also known as non-continuous, qualitative, or categorical (e.g. male or female, Gustilo type 1, 2, 3a, 3b, or 3c). These types of data can be analysed statistically using the chi-squared test or Fisher's exact test.

There are also continuous or variable data, e.g. age, height, ESR, knee valgus angle. These data often, but not always, occur in a normal or Gaussian distribution, e.g. a symmetrical bell-shaped curve.

Continuous data can be described using:

- 'Mean', which is the arithmetical average of the data set
- 'Median', which is the middle value of the data set when placed in ascending or descending order
- 'Mode', which is the most frequently occurring value of the data set

In a normal distribution the mean, median, and mode are equal.

'Dispersion' is the variability of a data set. If all the values were the same then the dispersion would be zero. There are various ways of measuring dispersion in statistics including quartiles, standard deviation (SD), and variance. For a set of data the range equals the lowest and highest numbers. The percentiles are groups of data in percentage brackets (usually 25%). The variance is a measure of how much a typical value deviates from the mean (variance = corrected sum of the squares about the mean). The SD is the square root of the variance (to give the same original dimension as the data) In a normal distribution 95% of values are within ±2 SD of the mean. The standard error of the mean (SEM) measures how closely the sample mean of the data set approximates to the population mean that data set was taken from. SEM = SD/$\sqrt{n}$.

Normally distributed data can be compared statistically using parametric statistical tests such as Student's t-test. Data which are not distributed normally require non-parametric tests.

What do you understand by the sensitivity and specificity of a test?

Sensitivity is:

- The ability of a test to detect cases that are positive
- It is equal to (all positive test results/all cases that are truly positive) × 100

Specificity is:

- The ability of a test to detect cases that are negative
- It is equal to (all negative test results/all cases that are truly negative) × 100

What factors do you look for in an outcome scoring system?

Accuracy = how accurate it is compared with a gold standard.

Validity = the extent to which an experimental value represents a true value (the usefulness or utility of a score or test).

Reliability = the ability to repeat the study/test and get the same results.

Ease of use = the assessment method should be appropriate and not too long, complex, or cumbersome.

Viva 38

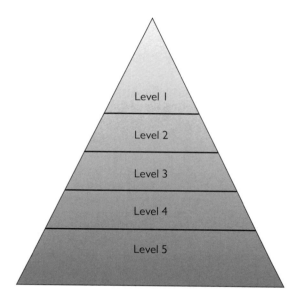

What is a systematic review?

What is a meta-analysis?

What levels of evidence do orthopaedic surgeons recognize?

What types of study do you know about?

What is the difference between bias and confounding?

What is the Cochrane Collaboration?

What is a systematic review?

A systematic review is an overview of primary studies that used explicit and reproducible methods.

What is a meta-analysis?

A meta-analysis is the mathematical and statistical analysis of the combined results of two or more studies that addressed the same hypothesis in the same way.

What levels of evidence do orthopaedic surgeons recognize?

1. High-quality randomized controlled trial (RCT)/systematic review
2. Low-quality RCT/prospective comparative cohort study/systematic review
3. Case–control study/retrospective comparative cohort study/systematic review
4. Case report or case series
5. Expert opinion

What types of study do you know about?

Descriptive studies:

- Case reports
- Correlational studies—studies which use large populations and correlate various factors to the presence of disease states
- Cross-sectional studies—studies which look at a particular group at one moment in time

Analytic studies:

- Studies where hypotheses can be tested, e.g. case–control studies, cohort studies, survival analysis, and interventional studies where a particular intervention is tested. The gold standard interventional study is the randomized double-blind clinical trial

What is the difference between bias and confounding?

Bias is a conscious or unconscious error in the way that cases are selected or measurements are taken in studies. It is often divided into selection bias and observational bias. Confounding occurs when factors not under study affect the results. The confounding factors may be linked to the factors under study.

What is the Cochrane Collaboration?

An International not-for-profit organization preparing, maintaining, and promoting the accessibility of systematic reviews of the effects of health care.

Viva 39

Item	Scoring categories
During the past four weeks	
1) How would you describe the pain you usually had from your hip?	1 None 2 Very mild 3 Mild 4 Moderate 5 Severe
2) Have you had any trouble with washing and drying yourself (all over) because of your hip?	1 No trouble at all 2 Very little trouble 3 Moderate trouble 4 Extreme difficulty 5 Impossible to do
3) Have you had any trouble getting in and out of a car or using public transport because of your hip? (whichever you tend to use)	1 No trouble at all 2 Very little trouble 3 Moderate trouble 4 Extreme difficulty 5 Impossible to do
3) Have you been able to put on a pair of socks, stockings or tights?	1 Yes, easily 2 With little difficulty 3 With moderate difficulty 4 With extreme difficulty 5 No, impossible
3) Could you do the household shopping on your own?	1 Yes, easily 2 With little difficulty 3 With moderate difficulty 4 With extreme difficulty 5 No, impossible

The picture above shows part of a questionnaire. What sort of questionnaire is this and when is it used?

What other ways are there of assessing outcome from surgery?

How might outcome measures be used in your practice?

The picture above shows part of a questionnaire, what sort of questionnaire is this and when is it used?

These questions actually come from the Oxford Hip Score, although these details are not as important as recognizing that it represents a patient-reported outcome measure (PROM). They are used for assessment of pre-operative pain and function and post-operative outcome.

What other ways are there of assessing outcome from surgery?

Several types of tool are available to describe outcome after hip surgery such as:

- General morbidity and mortality figures
- Generic quality-of-life questionnaires
- Disease-specific quality-of-life questionnaires
- Joint-specific outcome measures

How might outcome measures be used in your practice?

Outcome measures can be used to evaluate process outcome, including the performance of a surgical unit. They may also be used to evaluate a surgical procedure/prosthesis. The Department of Health now requires all patients undergoing joint replacement to have evaluation using the appropriate 'Oxford Score' to audit patient outcome. PROMs have become powerful tools in both clinical practice and clinical research.

Viva 40

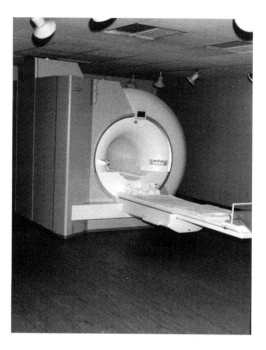

What is this?

How is it constructed?

How does it work?

What is this?

A magnetic resonance imaging (MRI) scanner.

How is it constructed?

It has three main components:

1. A superconducting electromagnet made of a niobium–titanium or niobium–tin alloy and cooled by liquid helium
2. A radiofrequency (RF) system consisting of a RF synthesizer, power amplifier, and transmitting coil
3. Gradient coils: these determine the positions of protons in the scanning field

How does it work?

1. The human body is composed mainly of water, which contains hydrogen nuclei (protons)
2. Protons align with the magnetic field in the MRI scanner
3. A RF pulse is applied, causing the protons to absorb some of its energy
4. When the RF pulse is turned off the protons release their energy as radio waves
5. The positions of the radio waves are determined by applying pulsed magnetic fields, using the gradient coils.

Viva Table 3

Trauma

Section 6 Lower Limb and Pelvic Trauma

Viva 41

This 27-year-old has been involved in a road traffic accident (RTA).

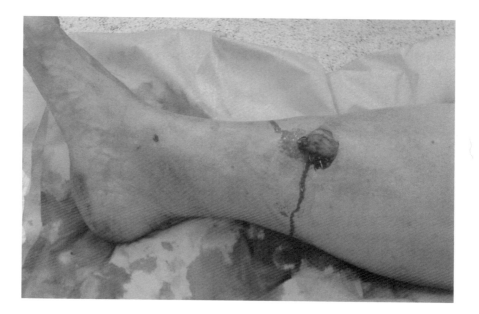

Describe what you see in this picture and explain your initial management.

When are you going to take this patient to theatre and what will you plan to do?

What is your biggest concern in the early post-operative period and how do you monitor for this?

How would you perform a lower leg fasciotomy?

How soon should you aim to get soft tissue cover and what do you know about free flaps?

Describe what you see in this picture and explain your initial management.

This is a clinical photograph showing an open fracture of the midshaft of the right tibia. After ruling out more urgent issues with an ATLS review, I would examine the wound, photograph it, and then cover it with a saline-soaked gauze. I would provide analgesia and splint the limb. I would give antibiotics and tetanus toxoid, if needed, and obtain AP and lateral radiographs.

When are you going to take this patient to theatre and what will you plan to do?

I would arrange for theatre at the earliest appropriate time (not necessarily <6 h). I would also discuss the case at an early stage with my nearest plastic surgical unit. I would perform an initial wash/scrub for gross contamination. I would then perform a thorough debridement of skin, fat, fascia, muscle, and bone. I would obtain fracture stabilization before further washout. I would apply dressings, splint the leg with the ankle plantegrade, and make a plan for future treatment.

What is your biggest concern in the early post-operative period and how do you monitor for this?

With any high-energy fracture, particularly tibial fractures, I would have a high index of suspicion for compartment syndrome. For this reason I would avoid regional anaesthetic blocks. In my unit we monitor patients with regular clinical observation. Invasive pressure monitoring is used for those patients who have a reduced level of consciousness.

How would you perform a lower leg fasciotomy?

I use the two-incision technique as described in the British Orthopaedic Association/ British Association of Plastic Surgeons (BOA/BAPS) guidelines published in 1997. The first longitudinal incision is 1 cm medial to the postero-medial border of the tibia and allows decompression of the posterior compartments. The second incision is placed 2 cm lateral to the anterior border of the tibia and allows access to the anterior and peroneal compartments.

How soon should you aim to get soft tissue cover and what do you know about free flaps?

The recommendation for definitive soft tissue cover is within 5 days of initial injury. Soft tissue coverage may be obtained by delayed primary closure or by one of the techniques of the reconstructive ladder. The most complex of these is the free flap. This usually involves taking a distant muscle with its vascular supply and revascularizing it with healthy vessels close to the recipient site. This muscle is then covered with a split thickness skin graft.

Viva 42

This patient was the driver in a high-speed RTA.

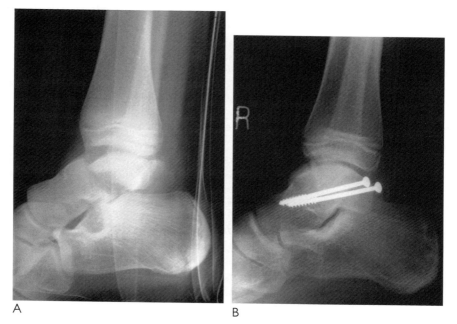

A   B

Reproduced from C. Bulstrode et al., Oxford Textbook of Trauma and Orthopaedics second edition, 2011, figure 14.11.3, p. 1717, with permission from Oxford University Press.

What do you see in this picture and what causes this type of injury?

What other information would you like?

What is the standard treatment for this fracture?

What complications should you anticipate in this patient?

What is the probability of AVN in this case and what would you see?

Can you describe the blood supply to the talus?

What do you see in this picture and what causes this type of injury?

This is a lateral radiograph showing a displaced talar neck fracture. The subtalar joint appears to be incongruent. I would classify this with the Hawkin's system as a type II fracture.

This injury is caused by the application of an axial load to the plantar aspect of the foot. This is a high-energy injury often associated with RTAs.

What other information would you like?

As this is a high-energy fracture I would be concerned about the general status of the patient and whether this was an isolated injury. I would want to have a full ATLS-type review. Regarding this injury I would want to know the neurovascular status of the foot and whether it was a closed injury. I would also require further radiographs of the foot/ankle and CT scan if available.

What is the standard treatment for this fracture?

Type II and III fractures should be reduced and fixed with two cannulated interfragmentary compression screws. I would use an antero-medial approach to the neck of the talus to openly reduce and fix the fracture from anterior to posterior. My aim would be for anatomical reduction as mal-union is associated with poor results.

What complications should you anticipate in this patient?

Early complications include compartment syndrome of the foot. There are a total of nine compartments in the foot. If necessary I would decompress the foot via two dorsal incisions, over the second and fourth metatarsals, and one medial incision.

Mid-term complications include infection, mal-/non-union, and AVN.

Long-term complications include osteoarthritis.

What is the probability of AVN in this case and what would you see?

Risk of AVN could be expected to be around 25% in this case. I would expect to see increased density of the talar body followed by subchondral collapse and talar dome fragmentation.

I would also look for Hawkin's sign. This is the presence of subchondral lucency seen radiographically around 2 months after fracture. It is a good sign, indicating reperfusion of the talus.

Can you describe the blood supply to the talus?

The blood supply to the talus is via an anastomosis formed by three main arteries and their branches. The predominant supply to the body is from the posterior tibial via the branch to the tarsal canal. The talar head and neck are supplied by the dorsalis pedis and artery of the sinus tarsi, a branch of the peroneal artery.

Viva 43

This rugby player landed awkwardly after a line out.

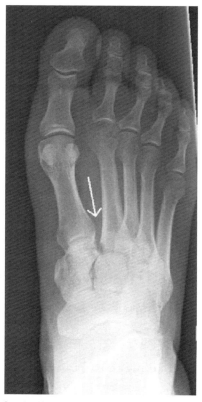

What do you see and which joint is involved?

What is the Lisfranc joint?

How do you describe Lisfranc injuries and which type is this?

This is an isolated injury. How would you proceed?

What do you look for on plain radiographs?

What is your operative plan for this fracture?

What are you going to say to this patient about his long-term outcome?

What do you see and which joint is involved?

This AP radiograph shows disruption at the tarso-metatarsal joints otherwise known as a Lisfranc injury.

What is the Lisfranc joint?

This consists of three cuneiform and two cuboid metatarsal articulations. Joint stability is provided by strong ligaments and the recessing of the second metatarsal head. The Lisfranc ligament runs from the base of the second metatarsal to the medial cuneiform.

How do you describe Lisfranc injuries and which type is this?

Type A is a complete uniplanar dislocation involving the whole joint. A type B injury describes a partial dislocation, either medial or lateral. Type C injuries are divergent dislocations.

In this case there appears to be a lateral type B injury.

This is an isolated injury. How would you proceed?

I would provide analgesia and elevation with a resting splint, including foot/ankle, but allowing room for swelling. I would observe for evidence of compartment syndrome and obtain further radiographic views and CT scan. I would wait for the swelling to reduce before considering surgery. Skin softening and wrinkling suggests that swelling is receding.

What do you look for on plain radiographs?

On an AP view the second metatarsal and medial cuneiform medial borders should align. On an oblique view the medial borders of the fourth metatarsal and cuboid should align. I would also look for the fleck sign which implies an avulsion of the Lisfranc ligament.

What is your operative plan for this fracture?

I would plan to openly reduce and fix with screws, starting with the second metatarsal reduction. I would employ two skin incisions, one over the first web space, the second over the fourth metatarsal.

What are you going to say to this patient about his long-term outcome?

I would warn him that even if his surgery goes well and things heal as planned there remains a 30% chance of post-traumatic osteoarthritis.

Viva 44

This 20-year-old roofer fell from his ladder sustaining this isolated injury.

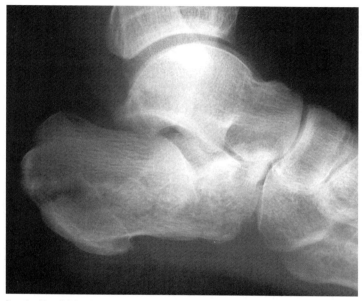

Reproduced from C. Bulstrode et al., Oxford Textbook of Trauma and Orthopaedics second edition, 2011, figure 12.61.9, p. 1419, with permission from Oxford University Press.

What do you see in this radiograph?

What is your management of this patient in the emergency department?

What further investigations would you order and how are these helpful?

How would you best treat this fracture?

Are you familiar with any published evidence in this area?

What do you see in this radiograph?

This lateral hindfoot radiograph shows a displaced calcaneal fracture with involvement of the subtalar joint. Bohler's and Gissane's angles are both reduced. Bohler's angle is normally between 20° and 40°; a reduction in this angle implies involvement of the posterior facet.

What is your management of this patient in the emergency department?

I would perform an ATLS review and look for associated injuries. More specifically I would assess the soft tissues and look for open wounds. I would assess and document the neurovascular status of the foot. I would then provide elevation and analgesia before obtaining plain radiographs of the calcaneum and foot. Clinical monitoring for signs of compartment syndrome would be commenced.

What further investigations would you order and how are these helpful?

I would like further radiographic views including Broden's views which help to visualize the anterior surface of the posterior facet. I would also request an AP view of the foot to assess the calcaneocuboid joint.

I would also request a CT scan. This provides a better understanding of the fracture configuration. CT also allows classification as described by Sanders. The Sanders classification of calcaneal fractures is based upon the position of the primary fracture line and the number of secondary fragments in the posterior facet.

How would you best treat this fracture?

The best treatment continues to be contentious. I believe that with good anatomical reduction, especially of the subtalar joint, outcome will be improved.

I would also discuss non-operative options and emphasize the potential risks of surgery. I would warn the patient that he is unlikely ever to have a 'normal' foot and that his career may well be affected.

Are you familiar with any published evidence in this area?

In 2002, Buckley et al. published a prospective, multi centre, randomized controlled trial [Buckley, R., Tough, S., McCormack, R., et al. (2002). Operative compared with non-operative treatment of displaced intra-articular calcaneal fractures. J. Bone Joint Surg. Am., 84,1733–44] which identified certain subgroups expected to have better or worse surgical outcomes. They studied over 400 patients with displaced intra-articular calcaneal fractures. Around 75% of these were followed up at between 2 and 8 years.

Overall the outcomes after non-operative treatment were not found to be different from those after operative treatment. Those patients, however, who were younger, female, or had an anatomical reduction scored significantly higher on the scoring scales after surgery compared with those who were treated non-operatively.

Viva 45

A 77-year-old woman fell off her bicycle sustaining this injury.

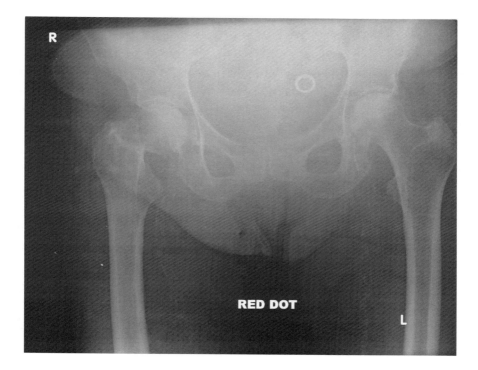

What does this radiograph show and how would you classify this fracture?

What would you like to like to know about the patient?

What is your initial management?

How would you manage this patient?

How would you manage this fracture if it occurred in a 42-year-old?

This patient presented at 10 p.m. Would you operate that night?

What does this radiograph show and how would you classify this fracture?

There is a displaced intracapsular fracture of the right neck of femur. I would describe this as a Garden IV fracture as there is complete displacement. Clinically the most important classification is simply between displaced and undisplaced fractures.

What would you like to like to know about the patient?

I need to know about any other injuries and the patient's acute medical status. I would then enquire about medical co-morbidities, residential status and her pre-morbid mobility. Her mental status both acutely and pre-injury are also important.

What is your initial management?

I would manage this patient along the recent British Orthopaedic Association Standards for Trauma (BOAST) guidelines. She requires analgesia, plain radiographs, and admission to an appropriate ward within 4 h. Routine bloods and electrocardiogram (ECG) are performed and the patient rehydrated. I would plan for surgery within 48 h unless a reversible medical condition was present.

How would you manage this patient?

As mentioned earlier, I would follow the BOAST guidelines. I would discuss treatment with her and propose a total hip replacement (THR). Studies show that patients do better functionally with THR and re-operation rates are lower. I would certainly expect this particular patient to do better with THR. I would use a cemented cup and stem with a 32 mm head via a modified Hardinge approach.

Although relatively uncommon, it is recommended that an orthogeriatrician should be involved in all phases of this patient's care.

How would you manage this fracture if it occurred in a 42-year-old?

I would aim to conserve the femoral head by reducing the fracture under direct visualization and fixing internally with three screws.

This patient presented at 10 p.m. Would you operate that night?

I would operate the next morning as evidence suggests that rapid surgery does not affect outcome. The most important factor is accurate reduction.

Viva 46

A 40-year-old sustained this injury in a RTA.

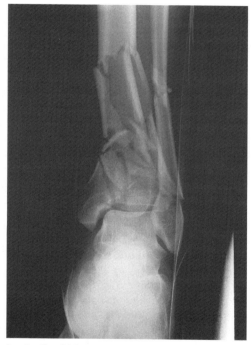

Reproduced from C. Bulstrode et al., Oxford Textbook of Trauma and Orthopaedics second edition, 2011, figure 12.15.4, p. 973, with permission from Oxford University Press.

Describe what you see in this picture and explain your initial management.

What is your primary treatment upon admission?

Do you know a way of classifying these fractures?

How would you definitively treat this fracture?

What are the AO principles?

What complications are you going to warn the patient about?

Describe what you see in this picture and explain your initial management.

This is an AP radiograph of the left ankle showing a multifragmentary pilon fracture.

I would perform an ATLS review and rule out concomitant injuries. I would then assess the neurovascular status of the affected limb and observe for signs of open injury or degloving. I would apply a temporary splint, provide analgesia, and obtain AP and lateral radiographs.

What is your primary treatment upon admission?

I would commence monitoring for signs of compartment syndrome. I would plan to take the patient to theatre and place a spanning external fixator. This would keep the limb out to length, maintain alignment, and most importantly avoid further insult to the soft tissues.

Do you know a way of classifying these fractures?

The Rüedi and Allgöwer [The operative treatment of intra-articular fractures of the lower end of the tibia. *Clin. Orthop. Relat. Res.*, **138**, 105–10, 1979] system describes three fracture types. Type 1 are essentially undisplaced, type 2 are displaced with little comminution, and type 3 fractures, like this one, have metaphyseal or articular comminution.

How would you definitively treat this fracture?

I would obtain a CT scan to enable pre-operative planning. I would consider discussing this patient with a specialist trauma centre. I would expect to wait around 7–10 days for the soft tissues to be in appropriate condition for surgery.

I would plan to openly reduce and fix along AO [Arbeitsgemeinschaft für Osteosynthesefragen] principles paying careful attention to the soft tissues. Non-surgical treatment is an option but would give poor results in this case.

Definitive external fixation would be a possibility, such as a fine-wire Ilizarov type frame.

What are the AO principles?

To appropriately restore bony anatomy, to maintain reduction while also respecting soft tissues, and to provide an environment that allows healing and early joint mobilization.

What complications are you going to warn the patient about?

Short-term complications I would discuss are: wound breakdown/infection, compartment syndrome, and chronic regional pain syndrome (CRPS). Mid-term complications would include non-union or malunion. I would warn that he is very likely to have long-term limitation of ankle movements. I would also warn that there is an 80% of developing post-traumatic osteoarthritis, although the symptoms from this may be variable.

Viva 47

This 26-year-old skier crashed.

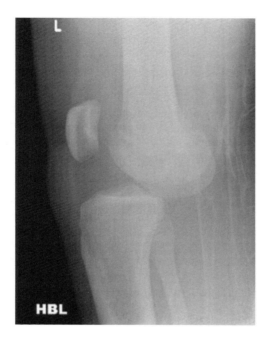

What does this radiograph tell you and what are your immediate concerns about the patient?

How do you carry out an initial assessment of this patient?

How do you classify these injuries?

This patient has an arterial injury—how will you proceed?

Which nerve is most commonly damaged and how would you manage this?

How do you provide definitive treatment for an unstable knee?

What does this radiograph tell you and what are your immediate concerns about the patient?

This lateral radiograph shows a dislocation of the left knee. This is usually a high-energy injury so I would be concerned about general patient status and other injuries. As far as this injury is concerned I would be most worried about a popliteal artery injury, which occurs in around 25% of patients with this injury.

How do you carry out an initial assessment of this patient?

I would assess and document the neurovascular status of the limb before reducing this dislocation, under sedation, as an emergency. After reduction I would again perform a careful neurovascular examination. If there is any suggestion of vascular injury, exploration or angiography is indicated. A 'normal' pulse may not exclude injury; an ankle–brachial pressure index of less than 0.9 is abnormal.

How do you classify these injuries?

These injuries are classified according to the direction of dislocation of the tibia in relation to the femur. Anterior dislocations are most common followed by posterior, lateral, medial, and rotatory dislocations. Up to 20% of knee dislocations have spontaneously relocated and do not, therefore, fit into this classification.

An alternative way of classifying is by description of the ligamentous damage incurred.

This patient has an arterial injury—how will you proceed?

I would arrange for this patient to go urgently to a theatre where a plastic or vascular surgeon will be available. Prompt reconstruction takes priority and would normally involve an interpositional vein graft. The knee would be stabilized, and thus the repair protected, by placing a spanning external fixator. Lower limb fasciotomies are also performed to avoid a reperfusion compartment syndrome.

Which nerve is most commonly damaged and how would you manage this?

The common peroneal nerve is the most frequently involved, occurring in around 20–30% of cases. I would treat this expectantly, although a large proportion will not fully recover.

How do you provide definitive treatment for an unstable knee?

I would obtain an MRI scan to characterize ligamentous structures that have been damaged. Associated fractures must also be sought. Additional information may be found by performing an EUA. Repair and/or reconstruction of ligamentous structures should be performed by somebody with experience in this area.

Treatment choices lie between early reconstruction of the postero-lateral corner (PLC) and posterior cruciate ligament (PCL), with delayed anterior cruciate ligament (ACL) reconstruction, and early bracing/rehabilitation with late reconstruction.

Viva 48

This young patient was the passenger in a high-speed RTA.

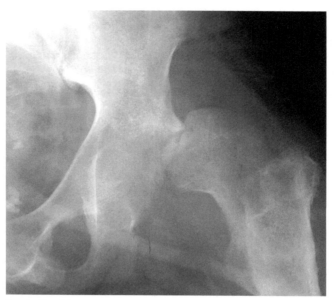

What does this radiograph show you and what would your initial management in the emergency department be?

Once in theatre how would you plan to treat this injury?

What would your management be once you have reduced the dislocation?

A CT scan shows an additional posterior wall fracture.

What are the indications for fixing the posterior wall fracture?

How would you fix this fracture and what complications would you warn the patient about?

What does this radiograph show you and what would your initial management in the emergency department be?

This is an AP radiograph of the left hip showing a posterior dislocation. There is an associated impacted fracture of the femoral head on the posterior acetabular wall. This is a high-energy injury and with a high probability of other injuries. I would therefore perform a full ATLS-type review. I would assess and document the neurovascular status of the limb and provide adequate analgesia. I would liaise with theatres and seek the advice from my local pelvic specialist centre.

Once in theatre how would you plan to treat this injury?

I would initially attempt a closed reduction of the hip. This is done using the Bigelow manoeuvre. With the patient supine and an assistant fixing the pelvis via the anterior superior iliac spines, the surgeon applies traction, adducts, and internally rotates the femur. The majority of dislocations will reduce with this manoeuvre. If the dislocation won't reduce then an emergency open reduction is indicated via a posterior approach.

What would your management be once you have reduced the dislocation?

I would confirm reduction on table with an image intensifier and perform an EUA to assess stability. I would place a distal femoral pin for traction to maintain hip reduction.

Post-operatively I would request further radiographic imaging including CT scan. This would confirm concentric reduction, rule out fragments within the joint, and characterize the posterior wall acetabular fracture. When the patient recovers from the anaesthetic I would repeat my neurovascular examination.

What are the indications for fixing the posterior wall fracture?

The indications for surgery are a lack of joint congruity or instability. Usually if only around 20% of the wall is affected the joint will be stable. Those with between 20 and 40% affected may or may not be unstable. In a young patient such as this, any involvement greater than 30% would be an indication for surgery to maintain reduction, and buttress plating will be required.

How would you fix this fracture and what complications would you warn the patient about?

I would use a posterior approach for this fracture. Screw fixation alone will be inadequate to maintain reduction and buttress plating will be required. I would warn the patient about early complications such as infection and sciatic nerve damage. Longer-term complications include heterotopic ossification (HO), AVN, and osteoarthritis. We routinely give indomethacin to reduce the risk of HO and give low-molecular-weight heparin to reduce the risk of DVT and pulmonary embolus.

Viva 49

This 32-year-old pedestrian was hit by a car.

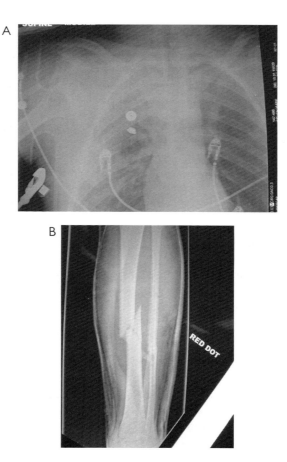

What do you see in these two radiographs?

What do you understand by the term damage control orthopaedics (DCO)?

How do you decide which patients require DCO and what is the alternative?

What is the Injury Severity Score (ISS)?

When do you expect to operate definitively on a DCO patient?

What do you see in these two radiographs?

There is an AP view of the lower left leg showing multifragmented mid-shaft fractures of the tibia and fibula, probably resulting from a high-energy impact. The chest radiograph suggests that there has been a significant insult to the chest/lungs.

What do you understand by the term damage control orthopaedics (DCO)?

DCO is a planned and staged surgical strategy in the management of polytrauma patients to minimize the effects of the 'second hit' on an already limited physiological reserve. The 'first hit' is from the injury and the body's response to this injury, while the 'second hit' is produced by surgical intervention.

Evidence shows that, in certain patients, primary external fixation of long bone fractures and secondary nailing improves outcome. There is a reduction in the incidence of multiple organ dysfunction syndrome (MODS) and adult respiratory distress syndrome (ARDS).

How do you decide which patients require DCO and what is the alternative?

The alternative way of managing polytrauma patients is known as early total care. This preceded the concept of DCO and involves the early treatment of all fractures. Patients who would be suitable for DCO include: those with Injury Severity Score > 20 with chest injury, those with abdominal or pelvic trauma in hypovolaemic shock (systolic blood pressure < 90 mmHg) and anyone with bilateral lung contusions.

What is the Injury Severity Score (ISS)?

This is a scoring system based on the Abbreviated Injury Scale (AIS). Each body system is given an AIS of 1–6 with 6 being the most serious. The ISS is calculated by adding the squares of the three most severely injured body systems. A patient with a score greater than 16 is defined as being seriously injured. In this case a patient would have greater than 10% chance of mortality.

When do you expect to operate definitively on a DCO patient?

This decision will be made in conjunction with the anaesthetist and intensivist. I would usually expect this to be after at least 4 days. Parameters such as blood pressure, heart rate, arterial blood gases, and core temperature must be corrected to avoid the risk of a large second hit.

I would want to exchange from external fixator to a nail within 10 days to avoid an increased risk of infection.

Viva 50

This woman fell while out shopping.

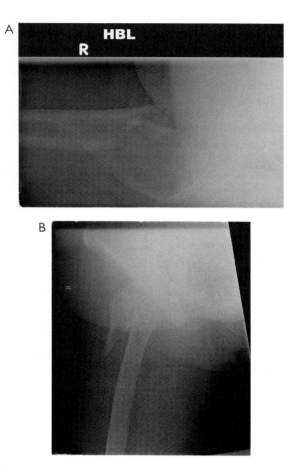

Describe these radiographs.

Who gets subtrochanteric fractures and how do you classify them?

How would you manage this patient in the pre-operative phase?

How do you fix these fractures?

When do you expect union and what is the risk of non-union?

Describe these radiographs.

These AP and lateral radiographs show a displaced subtrochanteric fracture on the right side. There is no evidence that this is a pathological fracture. Often in these fractures the proximal fragment lies flexed and in varus due to the unopposed pull of the iliopsoas. In this case the lesser trochanter has remained with the distal fragment so this deformity would not be seen.

Who gets subtrochanteric fractures and how do you classify them?

This is predominantly a fracture of the elderly. Although relatively uncommon, incidence is rising. Most are caused by simple falls from standing height. A significant portion of these fracture are pathological in origin. In young patients this fracture would invariably be due to a high-energy injury.

A universally accepted fracture classification does not exist. Classification is difficult because of different definitions of what constitutes a subtrochanteric fracture.

The Russell–Taylor classification divides fractures into four types. This classification describes piriform fossa involvement and medial buttress stability and acts as a guide to reconstruction.

How would you manage this patient in the pre-operative phase?

I would initially assess the patient's acute medical condition and exclude other injuries. I would then check neurovascular status, provide analgesia, and immobilize with a Thomas splint. I would obtain further radiographs including the whole femur. A thorough medical history is required as the association with metastatic disease is high.

How do you fix these fractures?

There is no gold standard fixation method for these fractures. Historically these fractures were plated, with nailing being a more recent option. All fixation methods have a sizeable failure rate which makes this a challenging area. The underlying problem is the massive biomechanical loads transmitted through this area.

For this particular fracture I would use a 95° dynamic condylar screw plate.

When do you expect union and what is the risk of non-union?

I would expect union to take around 4 months. This is a classic case of the race between fracture union and implant failure due to fatigue. Non-union risk would be in the region of 5–10%.

Viva Table 3

Trauma

Section 7 Spine and Upper Extremity Trauma

Viva 51

A 35-year-old man has been involved in a motocross accident and fallen off his bike. Wearing all the protective clothing and helmet he is brought into the emergency department complaining of neck pain.

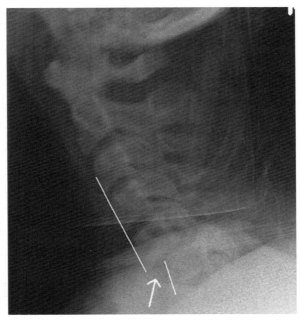

Reproduced from Aneel Bhangu, Caroline Lee, and Keith Porter, Emergencies in Trauma, 2010, figure 13.1, p. 268, with permission from Oxford University Press.

What are your comments about this radiograph?

How would you manage him now?

You don't have access to an MRI scanner; could you reduce this with the patient awake?

How would you apply a Halo?

What are your comments about this radiograph?

The C5 vertebra is displaced by 50% compared with C6, indicating a bifacet dislocation. This radiograph only shows down to C7 and is therefore inadequate for a trauma C Spine lateral radiograph.

How would you manage him now?

I would manage this patient following ATLS guidelines. I would initially remove the helmet visor to gain access to the eyes, nose, and mouth. I would then remove his protective equipment while maintaining spinal immobilization. One needs to exclude another spinal injury, and obtain full imaging of the spine. Having carried out a full neurological examination, and ensured that this is an isolated injury I would then contact a specialist spinal surgeon for advice on reduction. This can be a closed awake or open GA reduction. It is important to exclude a prolapsed disc which may damage the cord during reduction.

You don't have access to an MRI scanner; could you reduce this with the patient awake?

Yes you can, as long as the patient is awake, alert, and serial neurological examinations are possible. This is controversial. It is carried out by applying Gardner–Wells tongs to the skull and then adding sequential weights to the traction cord. The patient is supine, and an image intensifier is used to image the spine after each additional load is added. Ten pounds is added initially, and then approximately 5 pounds per level. Once the neck is fully stretched and the facets have been unlocked, the neck is then extended to complete the reduction, and the traction reduced.

How would you apply a Halo?

I would first explain to the patient how and why I am going to do it.

Four pins are used after local anaesthetic to the scalp, tightened with a torque limiter (six for a child). Placement is essential for:

1. Stability of the construct—equidistant and symmetrical
2. Prevention of damage to important structures—temporal artery/supraorbital nerves/sinuses

Placement is carried out as follows:

- Anterior—1 cm above lateral outer third of eyebrow (eyes closed)
- Posterior—behind earlobe above mastoid
- Three-person job—one holding the head and two applying the Halo
- Apply jacket—appropriately sized
- Check radiograph of the spine to ensure correct reduction is maintained
- Tighten the pins after 24 h

Complications include:

- Loss reduction/position
- Pin site infection and loosening
- Pain
- Nerve injury

Viva 52

A 35-year-old left-handed man sustained this injury whilst arm wrestling.

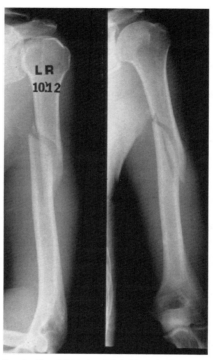

Reproduced from C. Bulstrode et al., Oxford Textbook of Trauma and Orthopaedics second edition, 2011, figure 12.11.8, p. 937, with permission from Oxford University Press.

Describe these radiographs to me. How would you go about managing this injury?

It is documented by the casualty officer that the patient has dense radial nerve palsy. How would this alter your management?

You've managed his radial nerve palsy expectantly, but after 4 months there has been no improvement. What would you do now?

What are the principles of tendon transfers? Which would you use here?

Describe these radiographs to me. How would you go about managing this injury?

These radiographs show an oblique mid-shaft fracture of the left humerus. My initial management would be to give the patient analgesia and a collar and cuff sling. I would take a mechanism of injury history and then examine the arm assessing the soft tissues (?open/?compartment syndrome) and distal neurovascular status (particularly radial pulse and radial nerve function). I would then take a more detailed general history—personality of patient.

You could treat this non-operatively with analgesia gravity traction in collar and cuff; however, I would have a low threshold for fixation in distal third fractures that are prone to slip into varus.

For operative fixation I would use a posterior approach:

- Position: patient on their side and the arm over a well-padded roll
- Approach: using a midline skin incision the plane is between the lateral and long head triceps—which is easier to find proximally (no true internervous plane, but muscles are innervated very high up so are not denervated). Look for the radial nerve and profunda A in the spiral groove coming medial to lateral—find/protect. I would then split the medial head in the line of fibres on to the bone (subperiosteal) more distally; beware the ulna nerve as it comes from the anterior compartment to the posterior compartment distally on the medial side
- Reduction and fixation: I would use a lag screw (large fragment set) and then a 4.5-mm broad DCP with four bicortical screws on each side (screws are offset)
- Closure: I would document the position of the nerve in relation to the plate

It is documented by the casualty officer that the patient has dense radial nerve palsy. How would this alter your management?

Treat radial nerve injury expectantly (90% are neuropraxias and recover within 3–4 months). Provide a wrist splint (in extension) for wrist drop/physio to maintain passive range of movement.

You've managed his radial nerve palsy expectantly, but after 4 months there has been no improvement. What would you do now?

I would organize nerve conduction and electromyography (EMG) studies. If these showed a neuropraxia, I would continue to monitor expectantly. If the muscle is denervated (axon or neurotemesis) muscle will show fibrillation potentials on EMGs (secondary to a hypersensitive post-synaptic membrane and random release of pockets of acetylcholine). I would refer to the local peripheral nerve injury specialist unit (wait at least 6 months).

What are the principles of tendon transfers? Which would you use here?

Tendon transfer is a late option, the principles of which are:

- A supple joint with full range of passive motion
- A healthy donor which is expendable, with grade 5 Medical Research Council (MRC) power (lose one grade with transfer), has adequate excursion, and is a synergist with a straight line of pull
- Good recipient site—tendon of paralysed muscle (if this is the reason for transfer)
- For a high radial nerve palsy common transfers include pronator teres to extensor carpi radialis brevis (ECRB_, palmaris longus to extensor pollicis longus (EPL) and flexor carpi radialis (FCR) to extensor digitorum (ED)

Viva 53

A 25-year-old man is brought into casualty with a closed isolated injury of his non-dominant right arm.

Can you describe the injury to me?

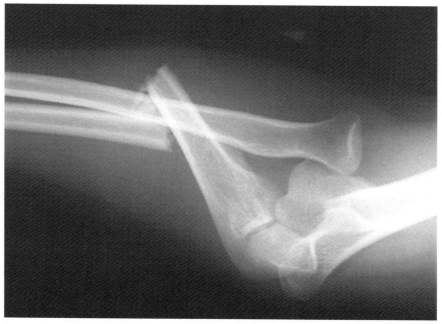

Reproduced from Aneel Bhangu, Caroline Lee, and Keith Porter, Emergencies in Trauma, 2010, figure 12.12, p. 234, with permission from Oxford University Press..

How do you classify these types of injury?

How would you manage this patient?

You choose to open and reduce the ulna fracture under direct vision and fix it with a dynamic compression plate. Tell me how this plate works.

Can you describe the injury to me?

This is an AP radiograph of the right elbow showing a Monteggia fracture dislocation. I would like to see further views of the whole forearm as well as a lateral view of the elbow to determine the exact direction of dislocation of the radial head.

How do you classify these types of injury?

Classification of Monteggia fractures is using the Bado system and is determined by the direction of radial head dislocation:

1. Anterior 70–85%
2. Posterior (5%; more common in adults than children)
3. Lateral (15–25%)
4. Any: with associated radial shaft fracture (rare)

How would you manage this patient?

Management of this isolated injury can be divided into initial A&E management and definitive management. I would first assess the patient in A&E giving some analgesia and taking a full history. On examination I would check the soft tissues for any evidence of open fracture or compartment syndrome as well as documenting carefully the distal neurovascular status. The posterior interosseus nerve is particularly at risk. This fracture dislocation needs to be reduced and fixed urgently. I would organize for the patient to go to theatre when medically safe. In theatre I would use a direct approach to the ulna shaft utilizing the internervous plane between extensor carpi ulnaris (ECU) (posterior interosseous nerve, PIN) and flexor carpi ulnaris (FCU) (ulnar nerve, UN). I would reduce the fracture under direct vision and then check with an image intensifier whether the radial head had relocated. I would fix this fracture with a 3.5-mm dynamic compression plate using AO principles.

You choose to open and reduce the ulna fracture under direct vision and fix it with a dynamic compression plate. Tell me how this plate works.

Compression can be applied across the fracture in a number of different ways. Firstly by pre-bending the plate; secondly by placing the screws eccentrically in the combihole to allow sliding compression at the fracture site; and thirdly by utilizing the compression device via a separately placed screw adjacent to the plate.

Post-operatively I would protect the soft tissues in a backslab for 4 weeks to prevent late subluxation of radial head. The patient would then require physiotherapy to regain elbow motion.

Viva 54

A 19-year-old rugby player presents to A&E with a first time injury to his dominant shoulder.

Comment on the radiograph.

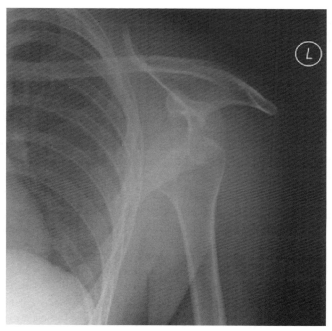

Reproduced from Philip G. Conaghan, Philip O'Connor, and David A. Isenberg, Oxford Specialist Handbook: Musculoskeletal Imaging, figure 4.6, p. 105, 2010, with permission from Oxford University Press.

Why does the shoulder dislocate? What stops it normally?

The A&E staff have tried to reduce this without success—talk me through how you would reduce this dislocation.

What is the risk of this shoulder causing problems again?

What approach would you do for an open reduction?

Comment on the radiograph.

This is an AP radiograph of the left shoulder showing an antero-inferior dislocation of the shoulder. One should look for associated injuries including greater tuberosity fractures, bony Bankart lesions and glenoid fractures.

Complications of anterior dislocation include axillary nerve palsy (5–30%), rotator cuff tear (14–63%, increased in elderly), greater tuberosity (GT)/glenoid rim fracture (>20%, = fixation).

Structures that may block reduction would include buttonholing through the capsule, biceps tendon, or bony fragments.

Why does the shoulder dislocate? What stops it normally?

The shoulder is a highly mobile joint, but at the expense of stability. When the restraints are overcome, the shoulder will dislocate. There are static and dynamic restraints.

Static restraints:

- Osseous anatomy limited to a third of the head on the glenoid—depth increased by labrum (~50%)
- Negative pressure inside joint
- Capsular thickenings—superior glenohumeral ligament (SGHL)/middle glenohumeral ligament (MGHL)/inferior glenohumeral ligament (IGHL) (most important—hammock analogy)

Dynamic restraints:

- Rotator cuff muscles
- Long head (LH) of biceps tendon

The A&E staff have tried to reduce this without success—talk me through how you would reduce this dislocation.

The patient has his arm externally rotated and abducted with loss of the deltoid contour. If the patient was still sedated I would attempt one further reduction in A&E. If unable to reduce I would mobilize my theatre team and anaesthetist to perform a reduction under GA:

- Hippocratic method—foot in axilla on humeral head, traction on abducted arm
- Kocher method of reduction—flex elbow 90°, arm in neutral, and then ER slowly until you hear a clunk of reduction. If does not reduce, flex shoulder, slowly internal rotate, and fully adduct across chest (no traction)
- Modified Stimpson—hanging weight prone

If the patient was young I would splint them in an ER position for the first 2 weeks then begin a mobilization programme guided by the physiotherapists.

What is the risk of this shoulder causing problems again?

The re-dislocation rate is proportional to the age at first dislocation.

There is a tendency to be more aggressive in the management of young, first-time dislocations. Use MRI arthrograms [look for Bankart (±bony)/capsular tear/Hill–Sachs lesion] or early EUA and arthroscopy to look for and repair Bankart lesions (labral detachment between 3 and 9 o'clock).

What approach would you do for an open reduction?

Deltopectoral. (See answer to Viva 2.)

Viva 55

A 30-year-old man fell off his mountain bike and presented to the emergency department complaining of shoulder pain.

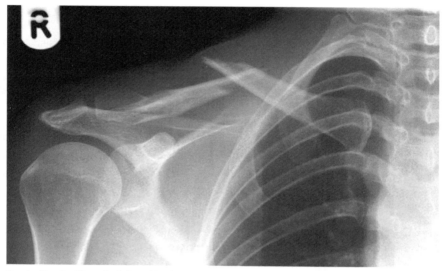

Reproduced from Aneel Bhangu, Caroline Lee, and Keith Porter, Emergencies in Trauma, 2010, figure 12.5, p. 217, with permission from Oxford University Press.

Describe the radiograph.

Do you know any classifications for such an injury?

How would you manage this patient?

Do you know any recent papers on the management of clavicular fractures?

Describe the radiograph.

The radiograph shows a displaced, angulated fracture of the middle third of the right clavicle.

Do you know any classifications for such an injury?

Clavicle fractures were classified into thirds by Allman [medial (<5%), mid (80%), lateral (15%)]. Neer revised the Allman classification scheme.

Lateral clavicle fractures were further divided into three types based on the location of the clavicle fracture in relation to the coracoclavicular ligaments:

Type I fractures occurred to the coracoclavicular lateral ligaments

Type II fractures occurred at the level of coracoclavicular ligaments, with the trapezoid remaining intact with the distal segment.

Type III injuries entered the acromioclavicular (AC) joint

The Neer Type II fracture was further divided into Type IIA, in which both the conoid and trapezoid ligaments remain attached to the distal fragment, and Type IIB, in which the conoid ligament is torn.

How would you manage this patient?

I would initially manage this patient on ATLS guidelines. He may have sustained a high-energy injury. I would ensure this was an isolated injury to the clavicle. Associated injuries include subclavian artery injury, brachial plexus injury, and lung injury. I would examine the neurovascular status of the upper limb, and the lung fields. I would assess the skin over the fracture. Most middle third fractures can be managed non-operatively, but this displaced shortened pattern has a higher incidence of non-union (10%), so I would openly reduce and internally fix this fracture with a pre-contoured plate.

Do you know any recent papers on the management of clavicular fractures?

Canadian Orthopaedic Trauma Society (2007). Nonoperative treatment compared with plate fixation of displaced midshaft clavicular fractures: a multicenter, randomized clinical trial. *J. Bone Joint Surg. Am.*, **89**, 1–10.

This was a RCT with 132 patients; non-operative vs operative midshaft clavicle fracture. The operative group had fewer non-unions (2 vs 7), fewer symptomatic mal-unions (0 vs 9), quicker time to union (16 vs 28 weeks), more satisfaction at 1 year. But the study was not stratified injury characteristics or subgroups.

Viva 56

Here is a radiograph of a child who has fallen off a swing.

Describe the injury to me. Can you classify it?

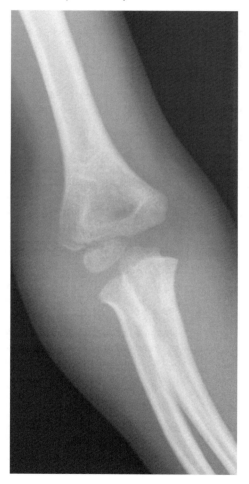

How would you estimate this child's age from the radiograph?

This is an isolated closed injury—how would you manage this definitively?

What are some of the complications of this particular injury?

Describe the injury to me. Can you classify it?

This is AP radiograph showing a displaced lateral condyle fracture.

Traditionally this injury is classified using the Milch system. This depends on whether the fracture exits into the joint relative to the trochlea. It has not been shown to be that useful in terms of guiding management. More important is whether the fracture extends into the joint.

How would you estimate this child's age from the radiograph?

I would estimate the age based on the fact that the ossification centres around the child's elbow appear in a standard order:

- Capitellum, 1 year
- Radial head, 3 years
- Medial epicondyle, 5 years
- Trochlea, 7 years
- Olecranon, 9 years
- Lateral epicondyle, 11 years

This is an isolated closed injury–how would you manage this definitively?

My definitive management of this injury would consist of open reduction of the displaced fragment and internal fixation to achieve absolute stability. I would hold my reduction with a partially threaded, small-fragment 3.5-mm screw. I would approach the fracture from the lateral side and check my reduction anteriorly avoiding the neurovascular posterior structures. Post-operatively I would protect the soft tissues in a backslab for 3 weeks, and then once they had healed I would start early range of motion exercises.

What are some of the complications of this particular injury?

These fractures have an unusually high rate of non-union for a children's fracture so interfragmentary compression with a lag screw is the optimum treatment. Other complications include angular deformity (cubitis valgus) secondary to a lateral growth arrest (more so in Milch Type 1 fractures). Management of such a deformity remains controversial. In my institution we would only consider an osteotomy at a later date if the deformity gave the child a functional problem. Tardy ulna nerve palsy is also a late, and luckily rare, complication.

Viva Table 4

Adult Pathology

Section 8 Foot and Ankle

Viva 57

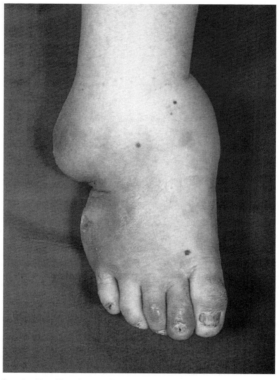

Reproduced from Murray Longmore, Ian Wilkinson, Edward Davidson, Alexander Foulkes, and Ahmad Mafi, Oxford Handbook of Clinical Medicine, figure 2, p. 205, 2010, with permission from Oxford University Press.

What do you see?

How does it evolve?

What are the principles of treating this condition?

What is this?

This is a clinical photograph of a grossly deformed foot and ankle.

Charcot arthropathy is a severe destructive arthropathy which can occur in any patient with a sensory disturbance. Over 90% of cases in the UK are related to diabetic neuropathy. (It occurs in 1% of diabetics who have had the disease for 12 years.) The other causes can be thought of along the course of the sensory neurological system from peripheral to central:

- Alcoholic peripheral neuropathy
- Post-traumatic sensory deficits
- Tertiary syphilis
- Spina bifida
- Hereditary motor and sensory neuropathy
- Congenital insensitivity to pain

How does it evolve?

The pathophysiology is not fully understood, but is generally thought to be due to a combination of both neurotraumatic and neurovascular factors. It is probably initiated by trauma; however, often no injury can be recollected by the patient. There is rapid destruction of the joint surface and demineralization, which appears to be a due to osteoclast overactivity, bone vascular shunting, and bone breakdown. This leads to loss of normal foot architecture. This phase is often said to be painless, but there is usually some pain (often less than may be expected). Healing begins and there is usually bony union with joint incongruity and foot deformity.

Eichenholz has staged this process:

- Collapse: the foot becomes painful, swollen (oedematous), and warm (erythematous). X-rays may show a fracture/fractures or dislocation. This stage can be difficult to differentiate from an acute infection. Over the following weeks the oedema and erythema settle, although the foot can continue to change shape (unless protected) as the bone continues to fragment. As a general rule, if the skin is intact think Charcot, if the skin is broken it is most likely infection, the history will often lead you
- Coalescence: the foot continues to settle and starts to stiffen up and the deformities become fixed. X-rays show coalescence of small fracture fragments and adsorption of fine bone debris
- Consolidation: over many months the oedema and erythema completely settle. X-rays show consolidation and remodelling of fracture fragments. (As a rough guide: forefoot 6 months, midfoot 12 months, hindfoot 18 months)

What are the principles of treating this condition?

1. Prevention: optimum management of co-morbidities (diabetes)
2. Early diagnosis: high index of suspicion, loss of protective sensation (use Semmes–Weinstein monofilament test, 5.02 monofilament)
3. In the early phase support the foot to maintain foot shape and prevent gross deformity. Weight bearing should be restricted. This must be done with care because patients often lack a protective sensation and casts and braces can cause ulceration (total contact casting)
4. Once consolidation is well under way the foot can be returned to some form of shoe wear (this can take many months, 12–18). Often life-long specially made orthotics will be required. Patients must be made aware of the risks of skin breakdown and inspect their feet closely each day

Viva 58

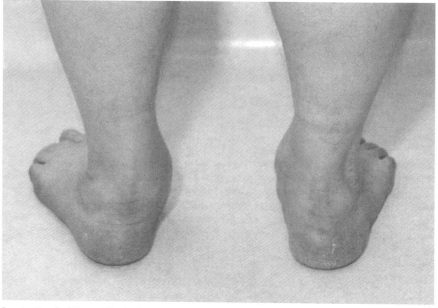

Describe this picture.

What are the stages of this condition and how are they managed?

Describe this picture?

This is a picture of a plano-valgus foot. There is the 'too many toes' sign. Pes planus can be congenital or acquired. The commonest cause of adult acquired flat foot is tibialis posterior tendon dysfunction (TPTD). The tibialis posterior is the main inverter of the hindfoot. It also acts as an elevator of the midfoot (sling) as it inserts into the navicular, plantar cuneiforms, and second, third, and fourth meta-tarsal (MT) bases.

The condition is most often seen in middle-aged women whose body morphology, aided by gravity, tests the tendon as it is starting to age.

What are the stages of this condition and how are they managed?

The tendon can become inflamed, painful, and swollen. The foot does not initially change shape and patients are still able to do a single leg tiptoe raise, although they quickly fatigue (Johnson Stage 1). Some patients settle with enforced rest in a supportive brace or cast.

As the tendon degenerates it lengthens. The foot changes shape with the hindfoot going into valgus. Patients are no longer able to do a single leg tiptoe raise. (Often the pain over the tib post may have settled, especially if the tendon has completely ruptured.) If the hindfoot is still flexible (Johnson Stage 2), this can be treated with orthotics to help support the foot and medial arch or by surgery. Surgery involves reinforcing the tibialis posterior tendon (TPT) with a flexor digitorum longus (FDL) tendon transfer. This reconstruction is then protected by bringing the hindfoot into neutral alignment with a medial sliding calcaneal osteotomy. The Achilles tendon occasionally needs to be released (percu-taneously), as if the hindfoot has been in valgus for some time it will have tightened preventing full correction to neutral.

If the valgus hindfoot deformity is fixed (Johnson Stage 3) reconstruction is not achievable. The sub-talar joint is degenerate. Surgical treatments involve a talo-navicular and subtalar fusion or a formal triple arthrodesis.

Myerson added a fourth stage when the deformity led to significant ankle arthritis secondary to valgus strain.

Viva 59

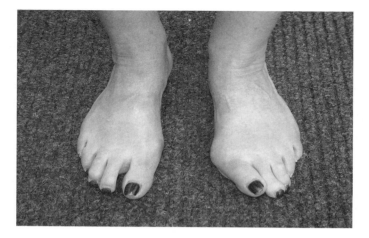

What is this?

What do you look at on the X-ray?

What are the treatment options?

What is this?

This is a clinical picture of a foot with hallux valgus (HV) and a large inflamed bunion.

- This condition is common
- Occurs in females four times as often as in males
- Most often in middle-aged women (also in teenage girls with a strong family history)
- Not common in parts of the world where no formal footwear is worn

Aetiology

There is a strong genetic component (FH +ve); inappropriate footwear plays a role.

Pathology

1. Capsule stretches medially
2. Structures tighten laterally (adductor hallucis)
3. Sesamoids stay with second MT attached via the intermalleolar ligament (IML)
4. MT head slips medially off the sesamoids via erosion of the crista and the hallux deviates laterally
5. Abnormal muscle pull of the extensor hallucis longus and brevis increases the deformity
6. As the first ray effectively shortens and defunctions patients begin to get transfer metatarsalgia. The second metatarsophalangeal joint (MTPJ) can become inflamed and synovitic, leading to clawing of the second toe and subluxation of the joint

Clinical symptoms

Pain due to the inflamed bunion; crossover of toes causing difficulty with wearing shoes; transfer metatarsalgia as the first ray defunctions; patients often complain of the appearance.

What do you look at on the X-ray?

Look at:

The severity of HV—HV angle (HVA) and intermetatarsal angle (IMA)

The state of joint and articular congruity, position of sesamoids

Second ray/subluxation of second MTPJ

HV interphalangeus (HVIP): IMA < 9°; HVA < 15°; interphalangeal angle (IPA) < 10°; distal metatarsal articular angle (DMAA) < 10° (discredited on most papers as not reproducible)

Sesamoid shift: grade 0–3 (0, none; 1, <50%; 2, >50%; 3, >100%)

Metatarsus prima varus = angle between long axis medial cuneiform and first MT

Natural cascade: first and second MTs same length; third 3 mm shorter; fourth 6 mm shorter; fifth 12 mm shorter

What are the treatment options?

Non-operative: information sheet; shoe wear modification (wide toe box); bunion pads and toe spacers; avoidance of high heels; analgesics

Operative: indications = failure of non-operative management or worsening pain (not for cosmetic reasons)

Surgical options are individual choices. In general if the IMA is <12 then a distal osteotomy may be acceptable (chevron preferred). If the IMA is >13 then a proximal or scarf osteotomy would be better. If the HV is marked (IMA > 20) or there is HVIP then an Akin osteotomy can be performed to give a more powerful correction. If there is osteoarthritis (OA) in the first MTPJ a fusion should be recommended.

Viva 60

This is a patient with rheumatoid arthritis.

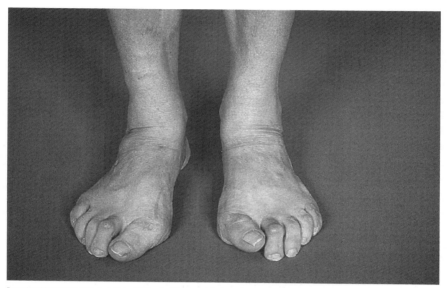

Reproduced from C. Bulstrode et al., Oxford Textbook of Trauma and Orthopaedics second edition, 2011, figure 10.2.3, p. 795, with permission from Oxford University Press.

What are the common deformities seen in the foot with rheumatoid arthritis?

How do these deformities occur?

Describe how you would manage this patient.

What are the common deformities seen in the foot with rheumatoid arthritis?

Rheumatoid arthritis (RA) commonly causes foot deformities. It can affect the forefoot, midfoot, and hindfoot. RA causes synovitis. The inflammatory response within the joint and the subsequent release of proteases and collagenases destroy hyaline cartilage and cause periarticular attenuation of soft tissue capsuloligamentous structures. This leads to instability and abnormal mechanics; secondary OA often leads to further deformity. The incidence of rheumatoid foot deformities has dropped dramatically with modern disease-modifying anti-rheumatoid drugs (DMARDs).

How do these deformities occur?

Forefoot deformity

1. Synovitis in the MTPJs leads to attenuation of soft tissues, in particular the plantar plate. Pain from the synovitis and disruption of the plantar plate allows the toes to claw up with hyperextended MTPJs and flexed IPJs
2. As the MTPJs sublux with disruption of the plantar plates (attached to the plantar fascia and fat pads which normally cushion the MT heads from direct pressure) the cushioning fat pads are pulled forwards
3. The MT heads become prominent in the sole of the foot—predisposing to callosities, skin ulceration and breakdown (feeling of 'walking on pebbles')
4. HV is often present but doesn't usually cause a problem

Mid foot deformity

Involvement of the midtarsal joint leads to collapse of the long arch. This can be secondary to failure of the TPT which normally acts as a sling for the midfoot.

Hindfoot deformity

Tibialis posterior insufficiency and gradual disruption of the talocalcaneal interosseous (IO) ligament (an important stabilizer of the subtalar joint) leads to progressive valgus deformity of the hindfoot and collapse of the medial arch.

Describe how you would manage this patient.

This would include a multidisciplinary approach. These patients have multiple other problems involving their musculoskeletal system as well as other co-morbidities. Often despite, considerable deformity, the feet may not be very disabling. In general it is sensible to address the more proximal joint problems first (hip/knee) It is important to work up RA patients prior to interventions as they have a higher risk of all complications—infection (~5%) and wound healing problems.

1. Medical optimization: multidisciplinary team meeting with rheumatologists regarding normal medication
   - Methotrexate to continue
   - Anti-TNF (plan surgery in between doses)
   - Decrease steroids as much as possible and dose peri-operatively
2. Anaesthetic input; cervical spine (flexion/extension views); positioning and padding
3. Other joints: upper limb function (difficulty with crutches/sticks), physiotherapy, and occupational therapy input

Management of foot disease

Non-operative management consists of: custom made orthotics to accommodate the deformity; padded heels; locked or limited motion ankle–foot orthotic (with valgus corrective T-strap); information sheets; medical optimization.

The goals of operative management are a stable pain-free plantar grade foot. The trend now is towards joint preservation. Historically the procedure was first MTPJ fusion with excision of lesser MT heads. Now consider scarf, Weil's, or Stainsby's procedures.

1. For HV: arthrodesis of MTPJ (10° dorsiflex/10° valgus)
2. Lesser toes, If the joints are destroyed, resection of MT heads (Fowler's) or proximal interphalangeal joint correction and fusion. If joints are OK and in a younger patient consider Weil's shortening osteotomy of MT heads which allows reduction of MTPJs and return of the fat pad into the sole of the foot
3. Midfoot: talonavicular fusion ± calcaneocuboid fusion
4. Hindfoot: triple fusion
5. Ankle: fusion vs arthroplasty (RA is one of the best indications for ankle arthroplasty as these patients are low demand and have other joints affected)

   - There are not enough data to indicate whether fusion or replacement is to be preferred for patients in whom either procedure would be an option
   - At ~10 years clinical success rates appear similar, with 70% satisfactory results after both procedures [Haddad, S.L., Coetzee, J.C., Estok, R. *et al.* (2007). Intermediate and long-term outcomes of total ankle arthroplasty and ankle arthrodesis. A systematic review of the literature. *J. Bone Joint Surg. Am.*, **89**, 1899–905]
   - The non-union rate for ankle fusion was 10% and arthroplasty survival rate 77% at 10 years

Viva 61

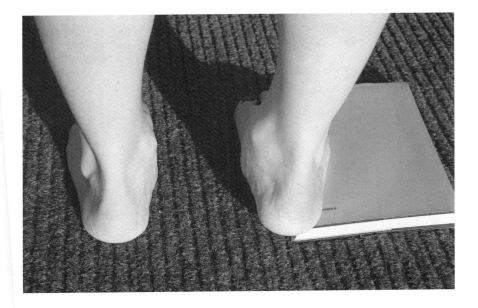

Describe what you see and how you would assess the patient.

What are the causes of this deformity?

How does a patient present and what are the principles of treatment?

Describe what you see and how you would assess the patient.

On inspection this patient has a varus hindfoot with a high medial arch or pes cavus deformity. The hindfoot deformity on the right is correctable with the Coleman block test. This shows that the subtalar joint is mobile and the varus hindfoot deformity is driven by excess plantar flexion of the first ray. I would expect there to also be clawing of the toes with hyperextension of the MTPJs and flexion of the interphalangeal joints. If this is unilateral it is due to a spinal cord tumour until proved otherwise. I would like to see the patient walk to check if they have a broad-based ataxic gait. I would like to have a look at their back and perform a lower leg neurological examination. I would inspect the hands for any intrinsic wasting. I would ask the patient what troubles they get from their feet so we can decide on a management plan.

What are the causes of caro varus foot deformity?

These can be congenital or acquired [hereditary sensorimotor neuropathy (HSMN) is the most common reason]:

Congenital: idiopathic; arthrogrypotic; residual clubfoot Acquired:

- Neurological: brain (Friedreich's ataxia)
- Spinal cord: spina bifida, polio, syrinx
- Peripheral nervous system: HSMN (Charcot–Marie–Tooth disease)
- Muscular: muscular dystrophies
- Traumatic
- Neoplastic

Charcot–Marie–Tooth disease/HSMN

There are lots of subtypes being described as the genetics improves, but there are two main types:
1. Early: Type 1, demyelinating type; autosomal dominant in 50% with six subtypes; ages 5–15 years; loss of reflexes; abnormal nerve conduction studies (NCS); hands involved
2. Later: Type 2, axonal autosomal dominant with 12 subtypes; ages 15–20 years; NCS are normal

How does a patient present and what are the principles of management?

Presents with deformity and instability, with repeated ankle sprains and painful callosities (secondary to clawing). History is important (is there a family history?).

Patients need a full assessment including: a neurological assessment, investigations—whole-body X-rays, MRI (spine), NCS ± EMGs

They should be referred to a neurologist for investigation of the cause and often a genetic consultation is helpful.

Orthopaedic treatment is best divided by the ability to correct the deformity:

Non-operative: stretching; physiotherapy; serial casts; in children ± orthotics [corrective, if flexible (e.g. lateral heel wedge) vs accommodative, if fixed]
Operative: soft-tissue or bony, or both

Aims of treatment are to achieve plantigrade, stable foot that moves and is pain free. Treatment decision is based on the age of patient and whether the deformity is flexible or fixed.

Viva Table 4

Adult Pathology

Section 9 Knee

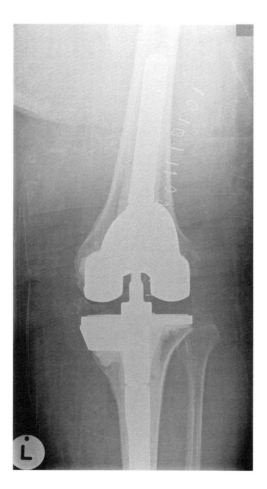

What implants do you use for revision total knee replacements?

[You are passed a hinged prosthesis] What are the benefits and disadvantages of this type of component?

If you were to revise a unicompartmental knee replacement what implant would you choose?

If you had a patient with a posterior cruciate ligament (PCL) sacrificing knee with a complete medial collateral ligament disruption and dislocation what implant choice might you make?

What implant do you use for revision total knee replacements (TKRs)?

[This question is aimed at exploring your understanding of pre-operative planning based on the individual requirements of the clinical case.] The range of implants or system I use would depend on the clinical situation: primary TKR, post stabilized, super-stabilized, rotating hinge, with stems ± augments, tumour prosthesis. Whenever faced with a revision situation it is also prudent to consider both amputation and arthrodesis as options.

[You are passed a hinged prosthesis.] What are the benefits and disadvantages of this type of component?

These implants are used in ligament insufficiency and/or cases with major bone loss. The problems with increasingly constrained implants are transmission of high forces across the bone–cement–implant interface which can lead to premature loosening.

If you where to revise a unicompartmental knee replacement what implant would you choose?

Ideally I would use a primary TKR implant. If there has been some tibial loosening and bone loss, a stemmed implant possibly with augments may be required.

If you had a patient with a posterior cruciate ligament (PCL) sacrificing knee with a complete medial collateral ligament disruption and dislocation what implant choice might you make?

Most likely I would require a rotating hinge stemmed system.

Viva 63

You see a patient 6 months following a right TKR. She is complaining of pain.

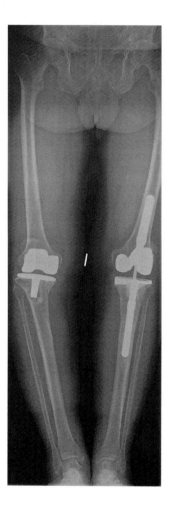

What are the commonest causes of pain following a TKR?

How would you investigate and manage this patient?

The blood tests show raised CRP and ESR, and the aspirate grows coagulase-negative, Gram-positive cocci after 5 days. How do you manage this?

What are the commonest causes of pain following a TKR?

This is still fairly early after a TKR and many patients still have pain that continues to resolve at this stage. Causes include:

- Infection—may not be commonest but is the most important to exclude
- Patellofemoral problems
- Component mal-position (overhang, mal-alignment, poor cementing)
- Loosening
- Complex regional pain syndrome (CRPS)
- Instability
- Dual pathology (hip arthritis)

How would you investigate and manage this patient?

Careful history: this needs to include an assessment of the patient prior to the TKR. The intra-operative and immediate post-operative care, including wound healing, length of stay, and any reported complications. Has there been a period when the knee was any good? How is the knee now (start-up pain)? Are there any co-morbidities—infection is more likely with diabetes mellitus (DM), RA, steroids

Examination: effusion/haemarthrosis, alignment, soft tissues, CRPS, ROM, PF tracking, patella clunk, balance, flex/extension mismatch, tender areas, hips.

Investigations:

- X-ray: component sizing, tibial overhang, femoral sizing, patello-femoral joint overstuffing, patella subluxation, loosening/infection, fractures, heterotopic ossification
- Blood tests: CRP, ESR
- Bone scan: no help at 6 months
- CT scan: may help assess rotation of components
- Aspiration/biopsy: if there is infection
- Arthroscopy: if a treatable cause is identified

The blood tests show raised CRP and ESR, and the aspirate grows coagulase-negative, Gram-positive cocci after 5 days. How do you manage this?

This seems to be a prosthetic infection with *Staphylococcus epidermidis*. I would discuss with the patient the diagnosis, the various treatment options, and the possible outcomes (function, further surgery, best- and worst-case scenarios). The treatment options would depend on the patient's physiological status and wishes:

Debride and retain

Revision (single stage or two stages)

Viva 64

A 25-year-old football player sustained a twisting injury to his left knee. He has already had an arthroscopy at 'St Elsewhere' and brings intra-operative pictures to show you.

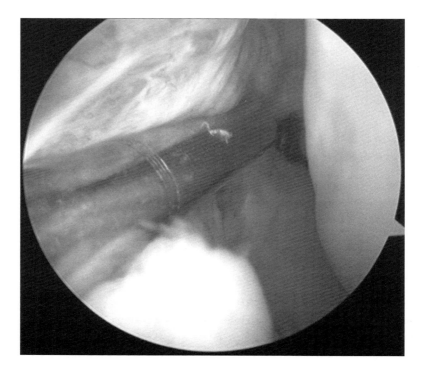

What does his arthroscopy picture show?

What is important in your initial assessment of this patient?

The patient now has recurrent instability and has been unable to return to sport. Your examination confirms an anterior cruciate ligament (ACL) injury and he has a full ROM. What are the management options now?

You have decided to reconstruct the ACL. What graft would you use?

What does his arthroscopy picture show?

The limited view shows a bare lateral wall of the femoral notch, in keeping with a complete ACL rupture.

What is important in your initial assessment of this patient?

The history of the injury, specifically how long ago

Symptoms since the injury: continued instability, locking, and significant subsequent injuries (is this an acute medial meniscus tear?)

Occupation and sporting aspirations

Expectations

Co-morbidities: diabetes mellitus, collagen disorder

Previous surgery

On examination: fixed flexion deformity; comfortable ROM; sign of meniscal pathology; signs of ACL disruption—Lachman and pivot tests (both can be negative in cases with bucket handle meniscal tears as the displaced meniscal tissue provides some increased stability to the knee); evidence of other ligament injury. If the patient has had significant secondary injuries it can be useful to get a fresh MRI scan to assess for secondary meniscal injuries.

The patient now has recurrent instability and has been unable to return to sport. Your examination confirms an ACL injury and he has a full ROM. What are the management options now?

There are two factors to address here: (1) treatment of the ACL and (2) treatment of any associated meniscal injury.

ACL injuries can be managed non-operatively and operatively. An assessment needs to be made of the risks of further meniscal injuries as this predicts the likelihood of early osteoarthritis.

Risk factors for high meniscal injury include: young age; level 1 sports; high number of hours participating in sport per week and previous meniscal injury. In view of this patient's history I would recommend an ACL reconstruction. The medial meniscal injury requires surgery. The key decision is whether to repair or resect the unstable meniscal tissue. Factors that would make you wish to repair the meniscus would be: recent injury (and easily reducible); red–red or red–white injury; concurrent ACL injury (increased healing rates); young age (it is also worth noting that the results of lateral meniscal repairs are better than those for medial meniscal repairs).

My choice would be to perform an arthroscopic ACL reconstruction and concurrent meniscal repair if indicated.

You have decided to reconstruct the ACL. What graft would you use?

[Have a view yourself.] I would use a four-strand hamstring graft with suspensory femoral fixation (EndoButton) and RCI screw fixation on the tibial side. But one should also be aware of the other options, as there advantages and disadvantages.

Autograft

- Hamstring tendons: good long-term results and low donor site morbidity but slower healing into bony tunnels
- Patella tendon: good long-term results, but donor site morbidity

Allograft

- Typically the Achilles tendon: no donor site morbidity but infection risk and, depending on sterilization techniques, less strong—and also expensive
- Artificial—avoid

Viva 65

This is a picture of a 67-year-old woman with a painful left knee. The pain has been increasing over the last 3 years. She is otherwise fit and well and has had previous joint replacements as shown.

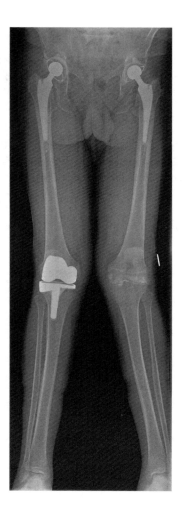

How would you manage this patient?

How would you consent the patient for a TKR?

Describe your plan for surgery in this case.

How would you manage this patient?

I would establish from the history more about her pain, disability, and what treatment she has so far received. On examination I would look at the nature of the deformity, whether it is correctable, the integrity of the medial collateral ligament, patella tracking, and neurological status (common peroneal nerve). I would examine her hip and foot. I would arrange some radiographs including standing AP, lateral. Von Rosenberg views and a skyline patella can be useful with valgus deformities. I may want a long leg film.

Treatment would include maximizing conservative measures. If this failed I would discuss with the patient knee arthroplasty surgery (lateral unicompartmental or total).

How would you consent the patient for a TKR?

I would describe the procedure as well as alternative treatments. I would describe the anticipated outcome in terms of pain relief; functional outcome, and longevity. I would explain the risks and complications of the surgery. General risks and specific risks for TKRs as well as specific risks for valgus TKRs.

Describe your plan for surgery in this case.

- Correct indications met
- Patient fully consented
- Antibiotic prophylaxis
- Choice of implant
- Choice of approach
- Principles of bony cuts, especially rotation of femoral component—how I will assess this (hypoplastic or wear on posterior lateral femoral condyle makes posterior referencing inaccurate)
- What I will do with the patella
- Soft tissue balancing (sequence of releases)
- Implantation of prosthesis and cementing technique
- Drain?
- Post-operative management and DVT prophylaxis
- Follow-up

Viva Table 4

Adult Pathology

Section 10 Hip

Viva 66

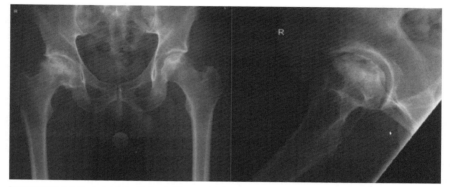

Reproduced from C. Bulstrode et al., Oxford Textbook of Trauma and Orthopaedics second edition, 2011, figure 7.16.1, p. 619, with permission from Oxford University Press.

What condition is illustrated here?

What is the aetiology and what risk factors are associated this condition? What other areas are commonly affected?

Can you describe any classification systems for this condition? What stage is shown in the radiographs above?

How would you manage a patient presenting with this condition? What treatment options are available?

What condition is illustrated here?

Avascular necrosis of the femoral head with segmental collapse.

What is the aetiology and what risk factors are associated with this condition? What other areas are commonly affected?

Osteonecrosis (avascular necrosis/aseptic necrosis) occurs within the bone following loss of osseous blood supply. All cells within the area of affected bone die away; initially the organic and inorganic matrix are unaffected. It commonly affects patients in the third, fourth, or fifth decades of life. The aetiology of osteonecrosis is still not fully understood and is likely to be multifactorial. Factors thought to contribute to the disruption of the microcirculation include:

- Trauma—leading to macro- and microvascular interruption
- Intravascular coagulation and thrombotic occlusion of microcirculation
- Extravascular compression ('compartment syndrome' within bone) secondary to raised intra-osseous pressures

Conditions associated with osteonecrosis include:

- Trauma
- Caisson disease (dysbaric osteonecrosis)
- High alcohol intake
- Systemic lupus erythematosus (SLE)
- Corticosteroid usage
- Ionizing radiation
- Haemoglobinopathy (sickle cell anaemia)
- Gaucher's disease
- Hypercoagulation disorders
- Idiopathic (40%)

Other areas most commonly affected are: medial femoral condyle; humeral head; talus; lunate (Kienböck's disease); capitellum (Panner's disease); tarsal navicular (Kohler's disease); metatarsal head (Freiberg's disease).

Can you describe any classification systems for this condition? What stage is shown in the radiographs above?

There are many classification systems described for osteonecrosis of the hip. The Ficat and Arlet (1980) system describes X-ray appearances and is one of the most simple to use:

Stage 1: no bony changes seen on plain X-ray
Stage 2: sclerotic and cystic changes within the femoral head
Stage 3: subchondral collapse and distortion of the femoral head
Stage 4: secondary osteoarthritis with decreased joint space and articular collapse

The radiographs show Ficat and Arlet stage 4 changes. There is distortion and collapse of the femoral head. The lateral view illustrates the 'crescent sign' associated with subchondral collapse.

How would you manage a patient presenting with this condition. What treatment options are available?

Treatment of early osteonecrosis of the femoral head aims to relieve pain and preserve the congruency of the hip joint. In the later stages of the disease arthroplasty procedures are usually required. Investigations used to help stage the disease include plain radiography, bone scans, and MRI.

Treatment for early stages (pre-collapse) may include:

- Observation and analgesia
- Treatment of any underlying medical conditions
- Protected weight-bearing (little evidence)
- Core decompression ± bone grafting or vascularized grafts

Treatment for later stages (post-collapse) may include:

- Realignment osteotomy
- Arthrodesis
- Replacement arthroplasty (conventional total hip arthroplasty or resurfacing)

Viva 67

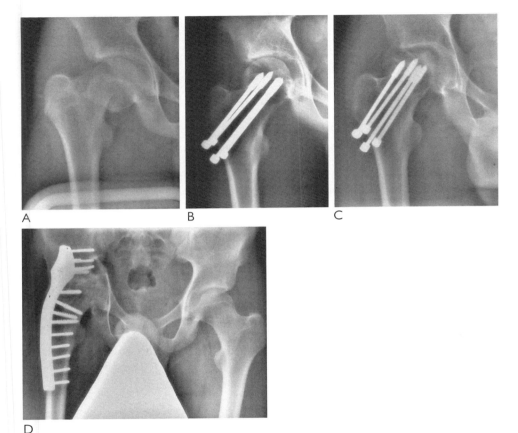

A   B   C

D

Courtesy of Dr S.L. Weinstein.

What considerations need to be taken into account prior to performing a hip arthrodesis?

In what position would you choose to arthrodese a hip?

What are the indications and pre-operative investigations you would perform prior to 'taking-down' an arthrodesed hip and converting to a total hip arthroplasty?

What considerations need to be taken into account prior to performing a hip arthrodesis?

Hip arthrodesis, although not commonly performed, is a useful procedure in the management of younger patients with end-stage unilateral hip disease who have contraindications for replacement or joint-preserving operations. Hip arthrodesis can provide long-term pain relief and stability to the joint. If performed correctly it can allow the patient to have a surprising amount of mobility and return to an active lifestyle.

Requirements for hip arthrodesis are:

- Normal contralateral hip
- Normal ipsilateral knee
- Normal lumbar spine
- No significant cardiovascular pathology

Long-term follow-up studies following hip arthrodesis have shown that the majority of patients develop lower back pain and ipsilateral knee pain 20 years or more after the fusion [Callaghan, J.J., Brand, R.A., and Pedersen, D.R. (1985). Hip arthrodesis. A long-term follow-up. *J. Bone Joint Surg. Am.*, **67**,1328–35]. The altered gait produced following arthrodesis has been shown to increase oxygen consumption by 32%—this may cause problems in patients with significant cardiovascular pathology.

In what position would you choose to arthrodese a hip?

The recommended position for hip arthrodesis is 20–25° of flexion, slight external rotation, and slight adduction. Internal rotation and abduction should be avoided. Care should be taken at the time of surgery to try and preserve the abductor muscle mass in case total hip arthroplasty is performed in the future.

What are the indications and pre-operative investigations you would perform prior to 'taking-down' an arthrodesed hip and converting to a total hip arthroplasty?

The indications to convert an arthrodesis to a total hip arthroplasty include:

- Increasing lower back pain/radicular pain
- Increasing ipsilateral knee pain
- Contralateral hip disease
- Painful pseudoarthrosis of the hip

Conversion of an arthrodesed hip to a total hip arthroplasty is a technically demanding procedure. Loss of the normal anatomical landmarks and supporting structures can lead to difficulty in restoring 'normal' joint stability and mechanics. The patient must be fully assessed prior to surgery. Investigations may include:

- Radiographs to assess bone stock and determine what metalwork (if any) needs to be removed
- Neurophysiology and/or MRI of the abductor muscle mass
- The potential for reactivation of dormant infection must be considered and appropriate biopsies taken pre- or intra-operatively

Viva 68

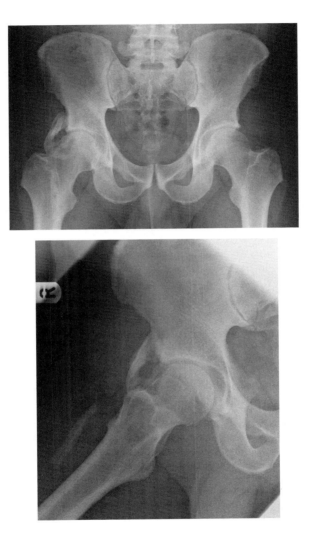

What do you understand by the term heterotopic ossification (HO)?

How can this affect patients clinically following hip arthroplasty surgery?

Are you aware of any risk factors for developing HO and what measures can you take to try and prevent this condition developing?

How do you manage established HO?

What do you understand by the term heterotopic ossification (HO)?

HO is the process by which mature lamellar bone forms outside the skeleton, usually in soft tissue. Causes include trauma, neurological injury, severe burns, and genetic conditions (fibrodysplasia ossificans progressiva).

How can this affect patients clinically following hip arthroplasty surgery?

HO following hip arthroplasty surgery is usually asymptomatic and noted as an incidental finding on post-operative radiographs. If the condition becomes severe it can present with restricted and/or painful movement.

HO is most commonly classified using the Brooker system:

Grade 1: islands of bone lie within the soft tissue around the hip

Grade 2: bony spurs protrude from either the femur or pelvis, with a gap of more than 1 cm between the spurs

Grade 3: gaps between the bone spurs are less than 1 cm

Grade 4: apparent ankylosis of the joint

Are you aware of any risk factors for developing HO and what measures can you take to try and prevent this condition developing?

Risk factors for developing HO around the hip include:

- Male gender
- Pre-existing hip arthrodesis
- History of HO in either hip
- Old age
- Ankylosing spondylitis
- Diffuse idiopathic skeletal hyperostosis
- Paget's disease
- Post-traumatic arthritis

Patients at high risk of developing HO or those undergoing surgery to remove HO are often given prophylactic treatment in the peri-operative period. The two main treatments available are NSAIDs and radiation therapy:

- Indomethacin is typically given at a dose of 25 mg three times a day for 5–6 weeks after surgery
- Low-dose radiation therapy may also be given, typically 7–8 Gy shortly before surgery or up to 72 h post-operatively

How do you manage established HO?

Management of established HO may be conservative or operative. Initial treatment usually involves physical therapy to try and improve mobility and range of movement in the affected joint. There is no evidence for the use of NSAIDs or radiotherapy in the management of established disease. Surgical excision may be performed if conservative measures fail. Most centres would advocate waiting until maturation of ossification prior to performing the excision (often > 6 months). Particular care should be taken at the time of surgery to clearly identify the neurovascular structures as they may be involved in the ossified tissue.

Viva 69

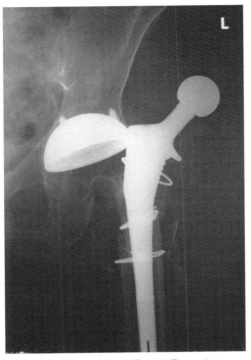

Reproduced from C. Bulstrode et al., Oxford Textbook of Trauma and Orthopaedics second edition, 2011, figure 7.10.4, p. 586, with permission from Oxford University Press.

What dislocation rate do you quote when you consent a patient for a total hip replacement?

What causes a hip to dislocate?

What measures can you take to prevent re-dislocation?

What dislocation rate do you quote when consenting a patient for a total hip replacement?

Dislocation following hip arthroplasty is one of the most common complications. Large studies have shown the incidence of dislocation following primary hip arthroplasty to be 3–5% over the life of the implant. The dislocation rate more than triples after revision hip surgery. The majority of dislocations occur in the first month (approximately 1%) and first year (approximately 2%). Over 50% of hips re-dislocate after initial closed reduction. Dislocation produces significant cost implications—both in terms of patient morbidity and the financial costs of treatment. It has been estimated that the cost of re-operation for a primary dislocation is 150% that of the original surgery.

What causes a hip to dislocate?

Causes of dislocation are multifactorial and can broadly be divided into surgical factors, patient factors, and implant design factors.

Surgical factors

- Component mal-position (most common)
- Soft tissue imbalance or failure of reattachment
- Soft tissue impingement (osteophytes/capsule)
- Retained debris (cement) in acetabular component

Patient factors

- Previous hip surgery or arthroplasty
- Female gender (relative risk 2.1)
- Acute fracture of proximal femur (relative risk 1.8)
- Inflammatory arthropathy
- Generalized soft tissue laxity
- Patient non-compliance (dementia, learning difficulties, drug/alcohol addiction)

Implant design factors

- Small head/neck ratios—leading to greater impingement risk
- Small head size (relative risk 1.7 with size 22 mm heads compared with 32 mm)
- Loosening of components leading to rotation and mal-alignment
- Wear of acetabular component leading to head subluxation

What measures can you take to prevent re-dislocation?

Prevention of re-dislocation can be attempted using conservative or operative methods. Assessment of joint stability should be made at the time of reduction. If the hip dislocates in the patient's normal functional range then it is likely that surgical intervention will be required.

Conservative methods

- Patient education, carer advice
- Physiotherapy and occupational therapy input
- Bracing of joint in an attempt to 'remind the patient' and prevent a position of instability

Surgical methods

Soft tissue laxity correction:

- Reattachment of avulsed soft tissues or trochanter
- Increasing neck offset using modular components

- Increasing acetabular lateral offset (lateralized liner)
- Trochanteric advancement

Increasing range of motion:

- Increase head–neck ratio (larger femoral head)
- Excision of osteophytes or soft tissues
- Increase excursion distance to dislocation (larger femoral head)
- Revision of mal-aligned components

Increase constraint:

- Augmentation of acetabular liners
- Constrained or captured liners

Viva Table 4

Adult Pathology

Section 11 Spine

Viva 70

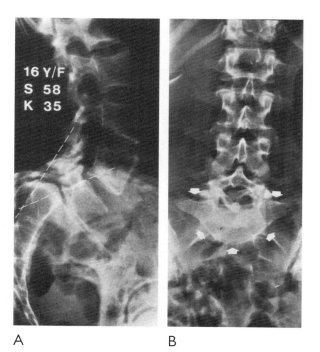

A   B

Reproduced from C. Bulstrode et al., Oxford Textbook of Trauma and Orthopaedics second edition, 2011, figure 3.17.6, p. 249, with permission from Oxford University Press.

What do you understand by the term 'isthmic spondylolithesis'?

What are the other recognized causes of spondylolithesis?

How would you grade spondylolithesis and what radiographic indices maybe used to predict progression?

How do degenerative litheses differ from spondylolysis when considering neural involvement?

What do you understand by the term 'isthmic spondylolithesis'?

Spondylolithesis is an anterior sagittal plane translation of a vertebra upon the adjacent caudal level. Isthmic spondylolitheses are secondary to defects in the pars interarticularis at that level. It is most commonly seen at the lumbosacral junction with defects in L5. The spondylolysis is considered to be secondary to mechanical factors leading to a stress fracture of the pars, often in sports delivering impact forces to the hyperlordosed lumbar spine in a genetically predisposed population.

What are the other recognized causes of spondylolithesis?

The other forms of spodylolithesis as described by Wiltse and Newman are Type I dysplastic, (Type II isthmic), Type III degenerative, Type IV traumatic, Type V pathologic, and Type VI iatrogenic.

How would you grade spondylolithesis and what radiographic indices maybe use to predict progression?

Meyerding graded lateral radiographs I–IV sequentially for each 25% slippage with spondyloptosis being a complete slip without endplate to endplate contact. Standing lateral radiographs can be assessed for pelvic incidence, sacral slope, pelvic tilt, and lumbosacral angle which have all been quoted as predictors of progression. Effectively all these parameters look at lumbosacral shear.

How do degenerative litheses differ from spondylolysis when considering neural involvement?

The striking difference is when the posterior elements are considered. In isthmic spondylolithesis the lamina of the affected level remains posteriorly placed and thus central and lateral recess stenosis are seen much less commonly than foraminal stenosis. In these cases a combination of degenerate disc and residual (cephalad pars interarticularis) and reduced foraminal height below the displace pedicle results in radiculopathy. This contrasts with degenerative slips where all three forms of neural encroachment can be seen resulting in a broader spectrum of symptoms.

Viva 71

A 67-year-old man falls onto his face and presents with an abnormal neurological examination and neck pain.

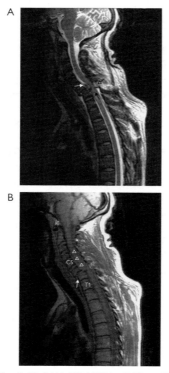

Reproduced from Hadi Manji, Adrian Wills, Neil Kitchen, Neil Dorward, Sean Connelly, and Amrish Mehta, Oxford Handbook of Neurology, 2006, figure 5.35, p. 399, with permission from Oxford University Press.

What do you see?

What is the most likely pattern of incomplete cord injury?

What are the clinical features of this injury and how would you manage the patient?

How do the clinical features of Brown–Sequard syndrome differ?

Are you aware of a grading system for cord injury?

How do you grade motor strength and test upper extremity myotomes?

What is spinal shock?

What do you see?

This is a T2-weighted sagittal MRI scan demonstrating Grade 2 spondylolisthesis of C6 upon C7 with large disc protrusion. The spinal cord is compressed and there is intramedullary signal change, in keeping with oedema, from C6 to T1.

What is the most likely pattern of incomplete cord injury?

Central cord syndrome.

What are the clinical features of this injury and how would you manage the patient?

There will be predominantly motor rather than sensory deficit affecting the upper extremity more than the lower extremity. It is not unusual to see marked early neurological recovery in such cases, and where no spinal instability exists non-operative management is the standard of care. However, in patients who plateau with a functional disability in conjunction with image-proven cord impingement surgical decompression and stabilization should be considered.

How do the clinical features of Brown–Sequard syndrome differ?

Cord hemisection characterized by: ipsilateral motor weakness, loss of proprioception and tactile discrimination, contralateral pain, and temperature and light touch deficit. There is anecdotal evidence to suggest somewhat better functional prognosis than central cord and anterior cord syndromes.

Are you aware of a grading system for cord injury?

The American Spinal Injury Association (ASIA) scale:

A = complete
B = sensory sparing/motor complete
C = motor sparing with >50% of muscle groups scoring <3/5
D = motor sparing with >50% of muscle groups scoring at least 3/5
E = no deficit

How do you grade motor strength and test upper extremity myotomes?

As described on the ASIA assessment sheets for neurological injury motor score grading (0–5):

0 = total paralysis
1 = palpable/visible contraction
2 = active, gravity eliminated
3 = active against gravity
4 = active against some resistance
5 = normal power for the individual

To test upper extremity myotomes: C5, elbow flexion; C6, wrist extension; C7, elbow extension; C8, long finger flexors; T1, finger abduction.

What is spinal shock?

A transient physiological state, characterized by loss of reflexes and sensorimotor function below the injury level. End of spinal shock is demonstrated by the return of the bulbo-cavernosus reflex (polysynaptic versus monosynaptic).

Viva 72

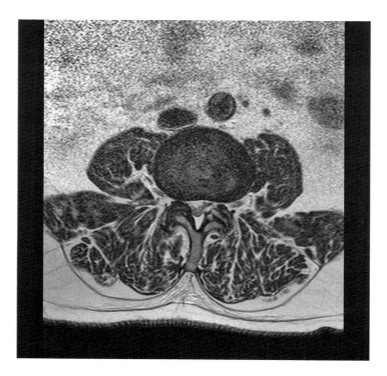

Describe the picture above and name the condition that is demonstrated.

What is the common clinical presentation for this condition?

Is there an anatomical classification for the condition?

What would be your indications for surgery in this condition?

When would you perform a fusion in this condition?

Describe the picture above and name the condition that is demonstrated.

This is an axial MRI scan (T2-weighted) at the L4/5 level that shows hypertrophy of the facet joints, hypertrophy of the ligamentum flavum, and a broad-based protrusion of the intervertebral disc resulting in severe stenosis of the canal, particularly in the lateral recesses. The condition is spinal stenosis.

What is the common clinical presentation for this condition?

The patient is usually middle aged or older and typically describes gradual onset of low back, buttock, thigh, and calf pain. They may also have numbness, pins and needles, or weakness. The symptoms are exacerbated by walking or even standing. A flexed position of the spine, e.g. pushing a shopping trolley, is often less painful than en extended position.

Is there an anatomical classification for the condition?

Degenerate spinal stenosis can be divided into:

Zone 1 or subarticular stenosis

Zone 2 or foraminal or pedicular stenosis

Zone 3 or extraforaminal or exit stenosis

What would be your indications for surgery in this condition?

Persistent significant pain despite adequate conservative treatment, including physiotherapy and analgesia. The patient should be fit enough for general anaesthesia and understand the risk of complications.

When would you perform a fusion in this condition?

The standard operation is decompression. Fusion should be considered in addition when:

- There is a significant spondylolisthesis
- There is progressive scoliosis or kyphosis
- There is removal of 50% or more of the facet joints
- There is fracture of the pars interarticularis
- There is radical excision of the associated disc causing possible anterior destabilization

Viva 73

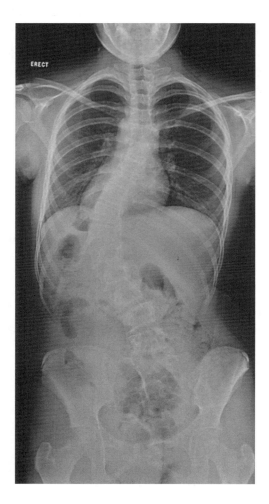

What is the name of the spinal deformity in the photograph above?

At what age and in which sex does it most commonly present?

What factors affect progression of the deformity?

How is it classified?

What is the name of the spinal deformity in the photograph above?

This is idiopathic scoliosis.

At what age and in which sex does it most commonly present?

It is commonest in girls and often presents around adolescence. The thoracic curve is usually right sided. The prevalence is around 3% of the population, although less than 10% of curves need treatment.

What factors affect progression of the deformity?

1. The future growth potential of the patient, i.e. the level of skeletal maturity at the time of diagnosis. This is measured by the Risser stage:
   - Risser 0 = no ossification of the iliac epiphysis
   - Risser 1 = 0–25% ossification
   - Risser 2 = 25–50% ossification
   - Risser 3 = 50–75% ossification
   - Risser 4 = 75–100% ossification
   - Risser 5 = fused epiphysis
2. The curve magnitude at the time of diagnosis:
   - Curves of <30° at maturity are unlikely to progress
   - Curves of 30–50° at maturity are likely to progress another 10–15°
   - Curves of >50° at maturity are likely to progress at around 1°/year
3. Sex: curves in females are more likely to progress
4. Curve type: double curves are more likely to progress

How is it classified?

There are two common classification systems.

King and Moe describe Types 1–5 depending on the shape of the curve:

- Type1: S-shaped double curve where the lumbar curve is larger or less flexible
- Type 2: S-shaped double curve where the thoracic curve is larger or less flexible
- Type 3: single thoracic curves
- Type 4: long thoracic curves where L4 is tilted into the curve
- Type 5: double thoracic curve where T1 is tilted into the thoracic curve

The more complex Lemke classification system describes the curve type (1–6) and adds a modifier (A, B, or C) depending on where the lumbar curve is in relation to central sacral vertical line, and another modifier (–, N, or +) based on the thoracic sagittal profile.

Viva Table 4

Adult Pathology

Section 12 Shoulder and Elbow

Viva 74

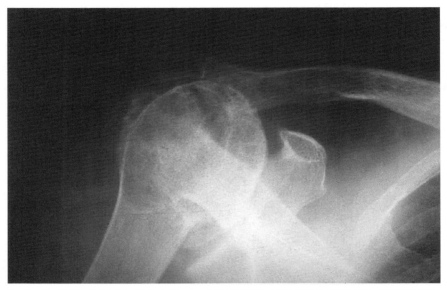

Reproduced from C. Bulstrode et al., Oxford Textbook of Trauma and Orthopaedics second edition, 2011, figure 10.3.6, p. 802, with permission from Oxford University Press.

Describe the radiograph. What is your diagnosis?

This is a 70-year-old fit and healthy patient with significant pain and stiffness. She has failed a trial of non-operative treatment. She wants surgery. What will you offer her? Explain how you would consent her.

What surgical approaches are you aware of?

If the patient had a massive cuff tear, what would you do?

Describe the radiograph. What is your diagnosis?

This is an AP view of the right shoulder showing a deformed humeral head with loss of joint space and subchondral sclerosis. This is osteoarthritis with a degree of avascular necrosis.

This is a 70-year-old fit and healthy patient with significant pain and stiffness. She has failed a trial of non-operative treatment. She wants surgery. What will you offer her? Explain how you would consent her.

I would offer her a shoulder hemiarthroplasty. I would explain to her that the procedure would not restore full movement in her shoulder, although the range of movement is likely to improve. The procedure is very good for pain relief. The procedure would be carried out under GA or regional anaesthesia. She is likely to stay in hospital for 2–3 days and will have to wear a sling for approximately 3 weeks and avoid external rotation to protect a repaired tendon (subscapularis). Her mobilization would be monitored by physiotherapists. The risks of the procedure include infection, injury to nerves and blood vessels, incomplete relief of symptoms, and implant loosening.

What surgical approaches are you aware of?

The procedure can be carried out through a Mackenzie (antero-superior) approach or a deltopectoral approach.

If the patient had a massive cuff tear, what would you do?

If the patient were to have a massive cuff tear, the outcome following hemiarthroplasty has been reported in the literature to be less satisfactory. This patient is unlikely to get any significant relief from non-operative treatments.

Counselling is needed before proceeding to hemiarthoplasty.

Viva 75

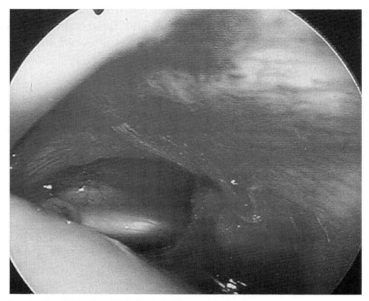

Reproduced from C. Bulstrode et al., Oxford Textbook of Trauma and Orthopaedics second edition, 2011, figure 4.5.1, p. 321, with permission from Oxford University Press.

What do you understand by the term 'frozen shoulder'?

What are the classical stages described?

What are the factors associated with this condition?

How would you manage this condition?

Are you aware of any operative procedures for this condition?

What are the typical findings during arthroscopy?

What do you understand by the term 'frozen shoulder'?

Frozen shoulder is the term used to describe the condition in which there is gradual onset of pain in the shoulder followed by stiffness.

What are the classical stages described?

The condition is typically characterized by three stages:

- Stage 1 is the painful phase which usually lasts 2–9 months. Patients usually complain of pain at night
- Stage 2 is the phase of stiffness and usually lasts 4–12 months. All movements are usually affected
- Stage 3 is the stage of thawing which also usually lasts 4–12 months. The stages overlap each other and are not discrete

What are the factors associated with this condition?

Factors associated with frozen shoulder are diabetes mellitus, trauma, chest disease, rotator cuff tear, hyperlipidaemia, and thyroid and autoimmune disease.

How would you manage this condition?

I would explain the diagnosis and natural history of frozen shoulder. I would offer an intra-articular steroid injection and analgesia, particularly in the painful phase. I would also refer the patient for physiotherapy. If symptoms fail to resolve, I would consider manipulation under anaesthesia.

Are you aware of any operative procedures for this condition?

Manipulation under anaesthesia by an experienced shoulder surgeon or arthroscopic capsular release is sometimes necessary for resistant cases.

What are the typical findings during arthroscopy?

The joint feels tight and the rotator interval is narrowed. Marked synovial injection is seen in the rotator interval.

Viva 76

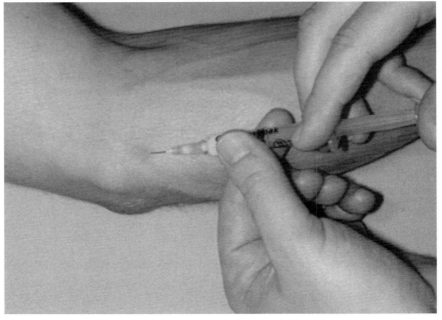

This figure was published in Orthopaedics in Primary Care, second edition, Andrew J. Carr and William Hamilton. Copyright Elsevier 2004.

What is tennis elbow?

What is the differential diagnosis?

What are the histopathological findings in this condition?

How would you manage this condition?

Describe the surgical procedure you would perform.

What is tennis elbow?

Tennis elbow is a condition characterized by pain in the region of the lateral epicondyle of the elbow. There is sometimes swelling and usually tenderness over the common extensor tendon. Resisted movements of the wrist and finger exteriors are usually painful.

What is the differential diagnosis?

Differential diagnoses include: cervical spine pathology; radio-capitellar osteoarthropathy, and radial tunnel syndrome/posterior interosseous nerve entrapment.

What are the histopathological findings in this condition?

A histological finding typical of this condition is angiofibroblastic hyperplasia, which represents a degenerative process. Extensor carpi radialis brevis is commonly involved and may have degenerative tears.

How would you manage this condition?

The management is mainly non-operative. I would advise patients on activity modification, analgesia, and use of a brace. I would refer them to physiotherapy. The role of steroids is being disputed— recent studies have shown no significant beneficial effect with steroids. Surgical release may be necessary if all non-operative treatments fail.

Describe the surgical procedure you would perform.

You should be able to describe the lateral approach to the common exterior origin.

Viva 77

A 19-year-old man participates in rugby at an elite level. He dislocated his left shoulder during a match 4 weeks ago. This was his first dislocation. It required reduction in A&E. He has no neurological problems and has regained full range of movement but his shoulder feels unstable.

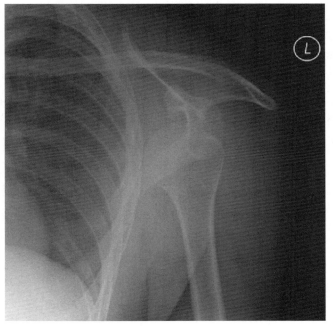

Reproduced from Philip G. Conaghan, Philip O'Connor, and David A. Isenberg, Oxford Specialist Handbook: Musculoskeletal Imaging, figure 4.6, p. 105, 2010, with permission from Oxford University Press.

What type of instability is he most likely to have?

How would you treat him?

What surgical options are available?

Describe the deltopectoral approach.

What type of instability is he most likely to have?

He has traumatic instability: this implies there is a structural defect—traditionally the TUBS classification has been used but now the Bayley triangle is most commonly used by shoulder surgeons and this case would be a Bayley Type 1 (traumatic, structural). A Bayley Type II is an atraumatic dislocation with a structural defect, while a Bayley Type III is habitual non-structural (muscle patterning). Placing patients in the correct group helps guide your management.

How would you treat him?

Surgically, he has had a significant traumatic event with a likely structural defect (the Bankart lesion). He is in a young age group, plays rugby at an elite level, and is at high risk of further dislocation. It is perfectly reasonable to proceed directly to surgery. It is reasonable to arrange an magnetic resonance arthrogram but some surgeons proceed to surgery based on the history and examination.

What surgical options are available?

A Bankart repair with inferior capsular shift. This can be done arthroscopically or through an open approach. The key stages are reattachment of the glenoid labrum between the 3 and 6 o'clock position on the right glenoid and the 6 and 9 o'clock on the left glenoid. At the same time an inferior capsular shift is performed which decreases external rotation. Physiotherapy is very important post-operatively.

Describe the deltopectoral approach.

See answer to Viva 24.

Viva Table 4

Adult Pathology

Section 13 Tumours

Viva 78

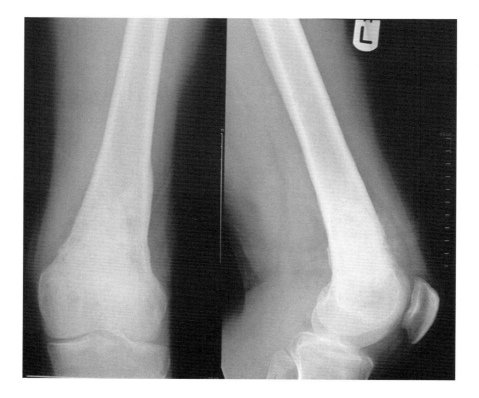

Describe what you see on these radiographs. What do you think is the most likely diagnosis?

How would you investigate this lesion further? What are the principles of performing an open tumour biopsy?

Outline your treatment options once the lesion has been identified and staged. Are you aware of any prognostic indicators?

Describe what you see on these radiographs. What do you think is the most likely diagnosis?

When describing bone lesions remember: age; bone; site; matrix; margin; periosteal reaction; soft tissue mass; likely diagnoses.

The radiograph shows a lesion arising from the distal femoral metaphysis in a skeletally mature patient

The matrix of the lesion is mostly sclerotic, suggesting osteoblastic (bone-forming) activity; there are also a few small lytic (bone destruction) areas

The margins of the lesion are not clearly defined with a broad zone of transition into the surrounding bone

The cortex of the bone overlying the lesion is poorly defined and has been invaded by the lesion

The periosteum has been elevated anteriorly (Codman's triangle) and there is an associated 'sunburst' spiculation appearance

The lesion appears to have expanded out into the surrounding soft tissues

These features suggest that this is an aggressive, fast-growing, osteoblastic lesion of the distal femur— the most likely diagnosis would be an osteosarcoma.

How would you investigate this lesion further? What are the principles of performing an open tumour biopsy?

Any bone lesion that is suspected of being aggressive or having malignant potential should be thoroughly investigated. Ideally these investigations and the subsequent management should be performed at a specialist tumour centre—early referral is recommended. Investigations are performed to accurately identify and stage the lesion prior to planning definitive treatment, these often include:

1. Local staging (performed prior to biopsy to prevent problems in interpretation):
   - Plain radiographs
   - MRI
   - Ultrasonography
2. Distant staging:
   - Chest X-ray
   - Computed tomography (CT) of chest
   - Bone scans
   - Positron emission tomography (PET)
3. Lesion identification:
   - Blood tests and tumour markers
   - Open biopsy
   - Tru-cut biopsy
   - Fine needle aspiration

The basic principles of open biopsy should be applied to prevent further seeding and spread of a potentially malignant tumour:

- The biopsy should be performed by the surgeon who will perform any definitive surgery
- No limb exsanguination
- The biopsy tract should easily removed with the incision for definitive surgery
- Utilize longitudinal extensile approaches, not transverse incisions
- Through compartments (muscle) rather than splitting through tissue planes
- No undermining of skin edges or tissue planes

- Adequate sample size and location—including the periphery of the lesion not just necrotic core tissue
- Immaculate haemostasis
- Drains brought out through or at the edge of the wound for easy tract excision

Outline your treatment options once the lesion has been identified and staged. Are you aware of any prognostic indicators?

Multi-agent chemotherapy in conjunction with surgery is the standard treatment for osteosarcoma. Typically neo-adjuvant chemotherapy is given prior to surgery. The tumour is then re-staged and definitive surgery is performed for local disease control—limb salvage (over 90% of surgery) or amputation options are available depending on the site and stage of the tumour.

Overall 5-year survival rates for osteosarcoma are approximately 60%. Patients with large-volume tumours, metastatic disease, or disease in the axial skeleton tend to fare much worse than those with peripheral and localized disease. Patients in whom a good histopathological response to neo-adjuvant chemotherapy has been achieved (>95% tumour cell kill or necrosis) have a better prognosis than those whose tumours do not respond as favourably.

Viva 79

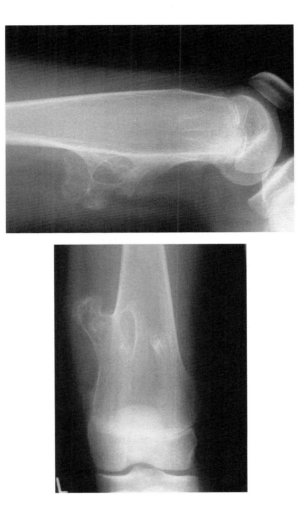

Describe the abnormalities you see on these radiographs. What is the likely diagnosis?

What is the inheritance pattern and natural history of this disease? What sites are commonly affected?

What clinical problems does it cause?

Describe the abnormalities you see on these radiographs. What is the likely diagnosis?

These AP and lateral radiographs show sessile lesions arising from the metaphyseal region of the distal femur. The lesions are well defined and appear to be growing away from the metaphysis. The matrix of the lesions is in continuity with the surrounding normal bone. The cortex of the normal bone appears to be in continuity with the lesions. The caps of the lesions contain flecks of calcification. These appearances would be compatible with a slow-growing, benign lesion, most likely osteochondroma.

What is the inheritance pattern and natural history of this disease. What sites are commonly affected?

Hereditary multiple exostoses (HME) is a familial inherited autosomal dominant condition but sponta-neous mutation also occurs. Males are more often affected, possibly due to an incomplete penetrance in females. Three gene mutations have been identified that can lead to HME. HME Type I is caused by a mutation in the gene encoding exostosin-1 (*EXT1*) which maps to chromosome 8q24. HME Type II is caused by mutation in the gene encoding exostosin-2 (*EXT2*), on chromosome 11, and HME Type III has been mapped to a locus on chromosome 19 (*EXT3*). There is some evidence for an additional multiple exostoses locus. The condition has an estimated incidence of 1 in 50,000.

Exostoses may be present at birth—over 80% of patients are diagnosed in the first decade of life (median age 3 years). There may be a few or hundreds of lesions present and the number and size tends to increase with growth.

The radiographic distribution of lesions is as follows:

- Distal femur 70%
- Ribs 40%
- Proximal tibia 70%
- Distal radius 30%
- Proximal humerus 50%
- Distal ulna 30%
- Scapula 40%

What clinical problems does it cause?

Generally, patients present with a painless mass. The developing exostoses may lead to abnormalities in osseous growth, joint restriction, joint deformities particularly affecting paired bones, and early progression to osteoarthritis.

Lesions that continue to enlarge after the end of puberty are abnormal and should be investigated for potential malignant change (chondrosarcoma). Ultrasonography and MRI are usually the investigations of choice.

Features suggesting malignant change include:

- Increasing pain and swelling (especially after cessation of normal growth)
- Thickening of the cartilage cap (>2 cm is very concerning)
- Lysis of a proportion of the stalk
- Intramedullary invasion of the underlying bone

Appendix

Diagrams for the FRCS (Tr.&Orth.)

Questions

There a certain number of diagrams that candidates get asked to draw—here are some that have been asked in the past

You should be able to sketch these out quickly. Try to talk and explain as you go so you are gaining points as you draw.

1. Draw and label a growth plate.
2. Draw and label the microscopic structure of muscle.
3. Draw and label the microscopic structure of cortical bone.
4. Draw and label a cross-section of nerve/tendon/meniscus/intravertebral disc.
5. Draw and label a cross-section of the spinal cord.
6. Draw and label a cross-section of articular cartilage.
7. Draw and label a proteoglycan.
8. Draw and label a stress–strain curve for bone/steel/titanium/plastic etc.
9. Draw and label the brachial plexus/lumbar plexus.
10. Draw and label the flexor/extensor tendon zones of the hand.
11. Draw and label a cross-section of the lower leg/mid-thigh level
12. Draw and label a screw used in orthopaedics.
13. Draw and label a cross-section through the vertebral column at L4/5.
14. Draw the graph of tibio-femoral angle from birth to adulthood.
15. Draw and label the zones around a total hip replacement.
16. Draw and label a graph showing how bone mineral density varies with age.
17. Draw out the pathways of calcium homeostasis/vitamin D.
18. Draw and label an inheritance table for an autosomal recessive/autosomal dominant/X-linked condition.
19. Draw and label a Z-plasty.
20. Draw and label a free body diagram of hip/elbow.
21. Draw and label a skeletal traction system that you know.
22. Draw a bacterium showing where antibiotics act.

Answers

1. Draw and label a growth plate.

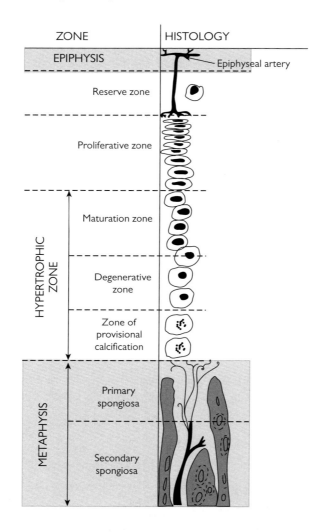

2. Draw and label the microscopic structure of muscle.

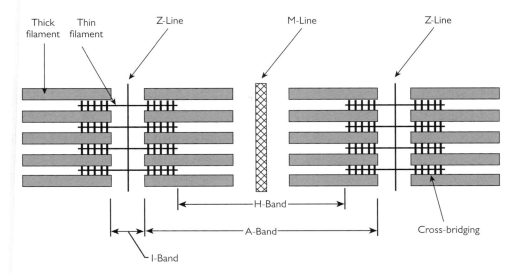

3. Draw and label the microscopic structure of cortical bone.

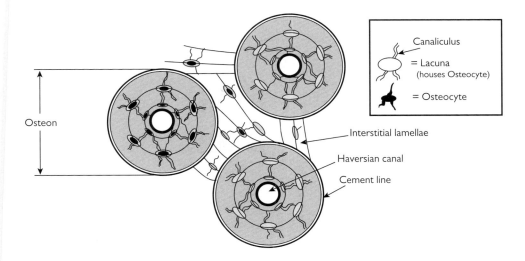

4. Draw and label a cross-section of nerve/tendon/meniscus/intravertebral disc.

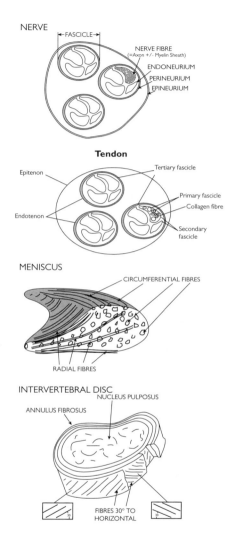

5. Draw and label a cross-section of the spinal cord.

POSTERIOR

Dorsal root ganglion

Dorsal columns

Dorsal root

Posterior horn

Lateral corticospinal tracts — Legs Trunk Arms

Grey commisure

Central canal

Lateral spinothalamic tracts — Legs Trunk Arms

Anterior horn

Ventral root

Ventral spinothalamic tracts

Ventral corticospinal tracts

ANTERIOR

Deep touch, vibration, proprioception

Pain, temparature

Light touch

Non-Decussating Sensory: <u>Dorsal tracts</u>
Decussating Sensory: <u>Ventral & lateral spinothalamic</u>
Motor (decussation in medulla): <u>Lateral corticospinal</u>
Decussating Motor: <u>Ventral corticospinal</u>

6. Draw and label a cross-section of articular cartilage.

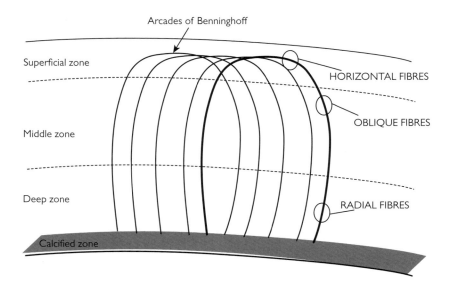

Arcades of Benninghoff

Superficial zone

HORIZONTAL FIBRES

OBLIQUE FIBRES

Middle zone

Deep zone

RADIAL FIBRES

Calcified zone

7. Draw and label a proteoglycan.

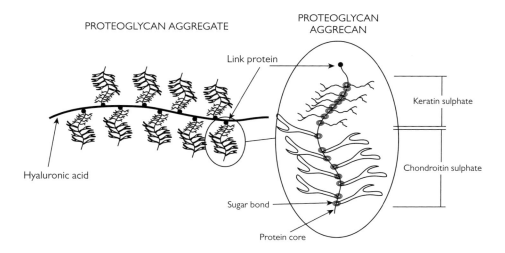

PROTEOGLYCAN AGGREGATE

PROTEOGLYCAN
AGGRECAN

Link protein

Keratin sulphate

Hyaluronic acid

Chondroitin sulphate

Sugar bond

Protein core

8. Draw and label a stress–strain curve for bone/steel/titanium/plastic etc.

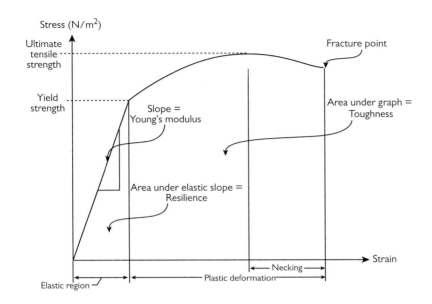

9. Draw and label the brachial plexus.

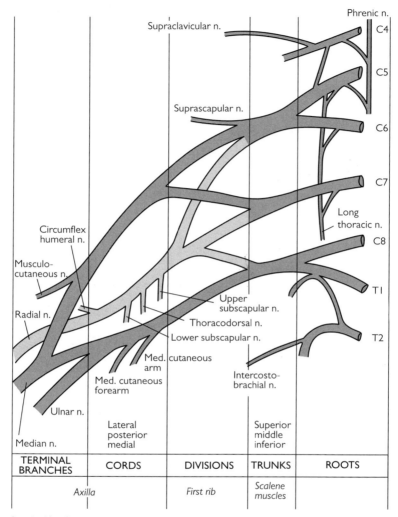

Reproduced from Graeme McLeod, Colin McCartney, and Tony Wildsmith (2012, forthcoming) Principles and Practice of Regional Anaesthesia fourth edition, figure 17.1, with permission from Oxford University Press.

10. Draw and label the flexor/extensor tendon zones of the hand.

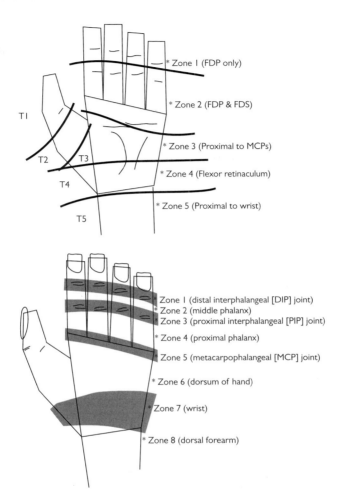

* Zone 1 (FDP only)

* Zone 2 (FDP & FDS)

* Zone 3 (Proximal to MCPs)

* Zone 4 (Flexor retinaculum)

* Zone 5 (Proximal to wrist)

T1
T2
T3
T4
T5

* Zone 1 (distal interphalangeal [DIP] joint)
* Zone 2 (middle phalanx)
* Zone 3 (proximal interphalangeal [PIP] joint)

* Zone 4 (proximal phalanx)

Zone 5 (metacarpophalangeal [MCP] joint)

* Zone 6 (dorsum of hand)

Zone 7 (wrist)

* Zone 8 (dorsal forearm)

11. Draw and label a cross-section of the lower leg/mid-thigh level

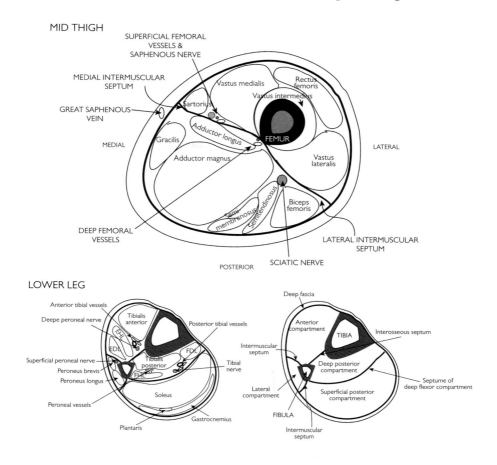

MID THIGH

SUPERFICIAL FEMORAL
VESSELS &
SAPHENOUS NERVE

MEDIAL INTERMUSCULAR
SEPTUM

Vastus medialis

Rectus
femoris

Vastus intermedius

GREAT SAPHENOUS
VEIN

Sartorius

MEDIAL

Gracilis

Adductor longus

FEMUR

LATERAL

Adductor magnus

Vastus
lateralis

Semi-
membranosus

Semitendinosus

Biceps
femoris

DEEP FEMORAL
VESSELS

LATERAL INTERMUSCULAR
SEPTUM

POSTERIOR

SCIATIC NERVE

LOWER LEG

Deep fascia

Anterior tibial vessels

Deepe peroneal nerve

Tibialis
anterior

Posterior tibial vessels

Anterior
compartment

TIBIA

Interosseous septum

Intermuscular
septum

EHL

EDL

FDL

Superficial peroneal nerve

Peroneus brevis

Tibialis
posterior

Tibial
nerve

Deep posterior
compartment

Septume of
deep flexor compartment

Peroneus longus

FHL

Lateral
compartment

Superficial posterior
compartment

Peroneal vessels

Soleus

FIBULA

Plantaris

Gastrocnemius

Intermuscular
septum

12. Draw and label a screw used in orthopaedics.

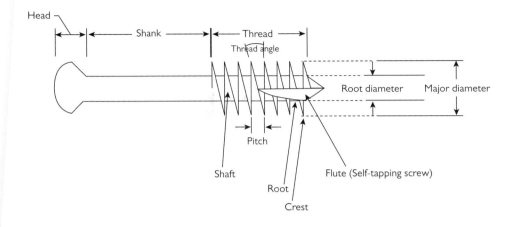

13. Draw and label a cross section through the vertebral column at L4/5.

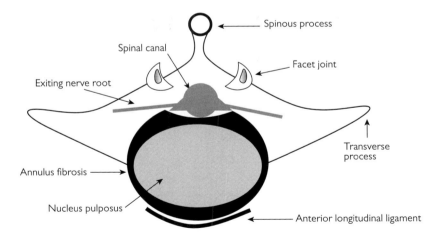

14. Draw the graph of tibio-femoral angle from birth to adulthood.

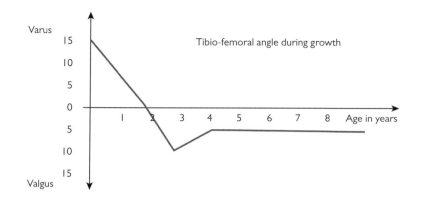

15. Draw and label the zones around a total hip replacement.

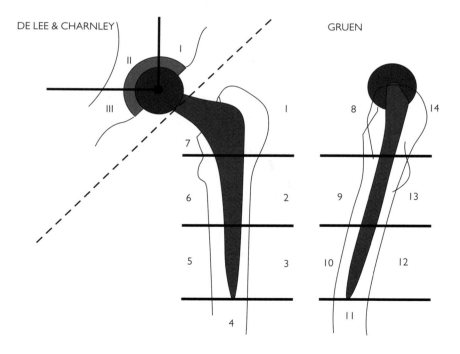

16. Draw and label a graph showing how bone mineral density varies with age.

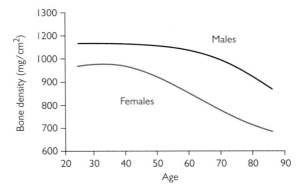

17. Draw out the pathways of calcium homeostasis/vitamin D.

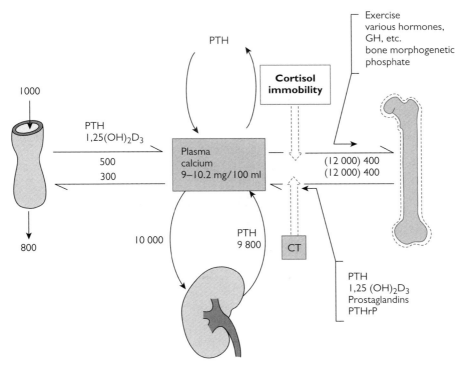

Reproduced from Smith, 1997, *Oxford Textbook of Rheumatology*, 2nd edition, Oxford: Oxford University Press, pp. 421–440, with permission.

18. Draw and label an inheritance table for an autosomal recessive/ autosomal dominant/X-linked condition.

AUTOSOMAL RECESSIVE

e.g. Friedreich's ataxia

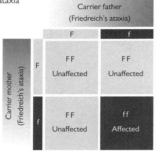

AUTOSOMAL DOMINANT

e.g. osteogenesis imperfecta
(Type 1)

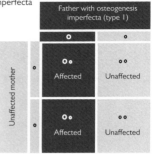

X LINKED

e.g. Duchenne muscular dystrophy

		Unaffected father	
		X	Y
Carrier mother (DMD)	X	XX Carrier daughter	XY Affected son
	X	XX Unaffected daughter	XY Unaffected son

19. Draw and label a Z-plasty.

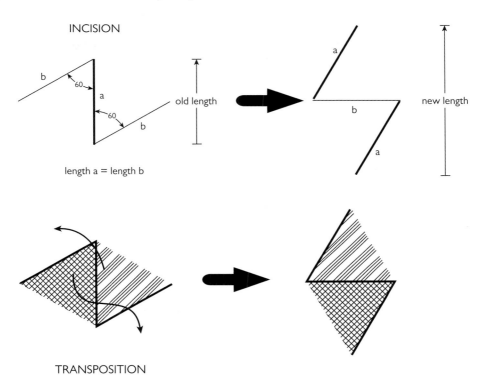

INCISION

old length

new length

length a = length b

TRANSPOSITION

20. Draw and label a free body diagram of hip/elbow.

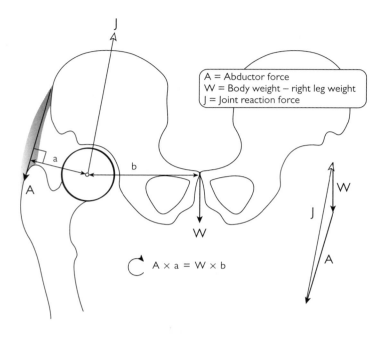

A = Abductor force
W = Body weight − right leg weight
J = Joint reaction force

$A \times a = W \times b$

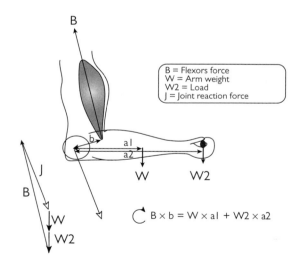

B = Flexors force
W = Arm weight
W2 = Load
J = Joint reaction force

$B \times b = W \times a1 + W2 \times a2$

21. Draw and label a skeletal traction system that you know.

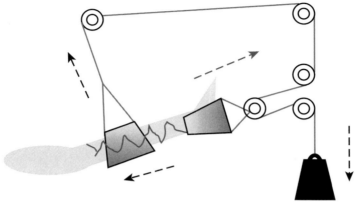

Hamilton Russell Traction

22. Draw a bacterium showing where antibiotics act.

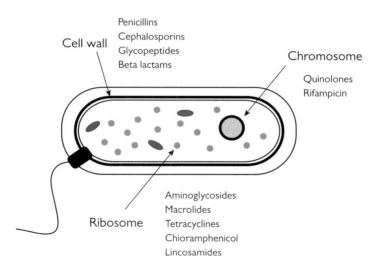

Cell wall
Penicillins
Cephalosporins
Glycopeptides
Beta lactams

Chromosome

Quinolones
Rifampicin

Ribosome

Aminoglycosides
Macrolides
Tetracyclines
Chioramphenicol
Lincosamides

Index

Note: page numbers in *italics* refer to figures.